ASPIRATIONS

my adventures with autism

VIRGINIA STA MARIA

Published by Vivid Publishing
A division of Fontaine Publishing Group
P.O. Box 948, Fremantle
Western Australia 6959
www.vividpublishing.com.au

NATIONAL
LIBRARY
OF AUSTRALIA

A catalogue record for this
book is available from the
National Library of Australia

Cover Photo by Manuel Goria
Illustrations by Virginia Sta Maria
Jacket Concept by Anna Johnson
Tiara Logo by Anna Johnson

ENDORSEMENTS FOR *ASPIRATIONS*

'A wonderfully quirky, at times humorous and always insightful book revealing personal characteristics, events, and reflections throughout Virginia's life. Thank you for letting the world into your colourful and fruitful life as an autistic girl and woman.'

Dr. Theresa Kidd, Clinical Psychologist & Author

'I came to know Oliver and Virginia Sta Maria and their son Aaron while coordinating the Curtin University Specialist Mentoring Program for neurodivergent tertiary students. Through their unwavering dedication, Aaron has been able to shape his best life going forward.

Virginia's courageous, autobiographical publication provides other families with the opportunity to understand and learn about a neurodivergent life from an insider, autistic perspective. She provides a raw, highly entertaining and poignant read that will entertain and educate a wide range of both neurodivergent and neurotypical individuals about the challenges of living a neurodivergent life.'

Dr. Jasmine McDonald BA DipEd MSpecEd(Hons) PhD.

'Virginia's book offers a deeply personal and moving memoir from the perspective of an individual with Autism Spectrum Disorder (ASD). Her candid narrative style provides a lens into her thoughts and emotions throughout different life stages. Virginia's book presents a heartfelt exploration of life with ASD, promoting understanding and connection for readers seeking to grasp the realities of individuals dealing with these experiences.'

Professor Tele Tan AM
Director, Autism Academy Curtin University

'Although written as an autobiography, this book is likely to have a more general impact on its readers by reminding them that during our life we all move along a mental health spectrum ranging from normal to psychopathological. The book also represents a personal contribution to a dimensional approach to Asperger's Syndrome by promoting its destigmatisation and humanisation.'

Aleksandar Janca, Emeritus Professor of Psychiatry

'Thank you so much for the privilege to read your book, Virginia. It made us blink away tears and laugh out loud! It is such a personal story. Knowing you, we can clearly hear your voice in our heads while reading. Your drawings are the icing on the cake! Readers of this book will quickly understand that:

- much can be told using bullet points
- it will take you into 'Aspie' thinking
- it is a humorous, admirable celebration of neurodiversity
- Virginia is a clever, funny, cool and beautiful inspiration for us all.'

Associate Professor Marita Falkmer
Emeritus Professor Torbjorn Falkmer

For Oliver and Aaron

With you guys in my life, everything is possible.

FOREWORD

I first met Virginia in 2014 when she attended my clinic for a psychological assessment along with her husband, Oliver. That interview impressed me in several ways. I can still recall the examples of abuse and neglect Virginia endured as a child. If she was not as 'matter of fact' in her mindset as she is, she probably would not have survived that extent of life adversity. Despite the heart-wrenching recalls, the interview room would sometimes roar with laughter because Virginia just has a way of saying things lucidly yet amusingly.

I could see she was genuinely admired by Oliver, who had seen beyond the social gaucherie to recognise her compassionate, upright, and loyal soul. Virginia, on the other hand, highly regarded Oliver as her social sight. It was touching to witness, within this neurodiverse relationship, an appreciation that was beyond acceptance.

It was not hard for me to identify the profile of Autism Spectrum Disorder (ASD) in Virginia. Her worldview made good sense to me when I put on the autistic lens. For instance, her 'off on a tangent' conversation style was owing to a literal mindset; her offensive comments at family gatherings stemmed from a strong sense of social justice; her pedanticism was due to an unusual capacity for details; her 'tantrums' a result of sensory overload and so on.

Virginia's candour, her firsthand experience in an autistic world and her remarkable autobiographical memory, prompted me to encourage her to share her worldview through a book.

I regard this an informative-comical-autobiography. This book tells you about Virginia's life journey, teaches you about an autistic worldview, gives you some belly laughs and, possibly, turns on a few light bulbs about human for you. Like the world of many autistic individuals, this book is full of contradictions.

First, many of the stories are hilarious yet sobering. They elucidate the vulnerability of an autistic person living in a non-autistic world. Second, you can see that Virginia is remarkably intelligent, yet she is unwitting in so many aspects of life. Third, the illustrations are ingenuous but telling. I encourage you to pause and ponder on the implications of Virginia's encounters. And finally, the presentation of this book is childlike but oh boy you will get some uncensored information!

This book is exceptional for another reason: it is an autistic friendly book written by an autistic person. The succinct illustrations conveyed through words as well as visuals make this book suitable for readers who are visual thinkers, tend to interpret words literally, have short attention spans and have negative associations with reading. Having worked with the autistic population for the past two decades, I deeply appreciate having a book that caters for people who find processing text challenging.

Virginia, being a childhood abuse fighter, a justice ambassador, a devoted wife and mother and now an author, should be proud of herself.

Dr. Winnie Yu Pow Blake (nee Lau)

Clinical Psychologist

INTRODUCTION

by Virginia Sta Maria

- At the age of 49, after years of wondering why I didn't fit in with the rest of the world, I was diagnosed with Asperger's Syndrome.

- Although the syndrome was redefined in 2013 as Autism Spectrum Disorder, I like the term Asperger's or Aspie for short and that is why I have used it in my book. My husband, Oliver, said 'It's because you are old.' I agree.

- I wanted to write a book because I am a person who loves to learn, and I am amazed that after speaking with many fellow Aspergian people I have knowledge I can share.

- Writing this book has shown me how socially blind I can be. I just can't see what is going on around me. When my husband Oliver explains things to me, I can then see, and it seems so simple, but at the time I am blind to the situation. My brain is just not wired that way. I am not wired for social.

- I have come a long way with learning how to socialise. I feel I have learned enough formulas, but I still find socialising stressful if I can't prepare.

- To other people, I just seem unusual in the things I say and do but they do not know how hard my brain is working. It is not easy to live in a non-autistic world where a massive part of life (socialising) is not natural to me.

- In my life I seem to make a lot of people angry with me when I am just trying to understand what is going on.

- I chose to use boxes, bullet points and illustrations for this book. My style makes it more reader-friendly where big chunks of text can be overwhelming to take in. The boxes are emotional, not cosmetic - I feel the boxes, the boxes give me structure.

- Using personal stories helps people reflect on their own experiences, so that they can say to themselves, 'Hey, I do that!'

- My 'Thinking Back' segments show people that things can be worked out, that there are different ways of thinking about things that happen.

- My 'Reading Faces' segments illustrate how I have totally misread the faces that other people pull. I can see that their face is different but do not know why, and as you will see, my guesses are quite original.

- Even though some of my pages may seem distressing, I just see them as interesting. I wrote about how I worked things out and my thought processes at the time, and now, as I look back, I can't help seeing the funny side.

- My hope for this book is that it will reach others like me who struggle with the ups and downs of autism, and those who want to learn more about what it's really like to experience it.

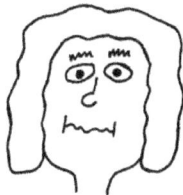

'Asperger's syndrome : an autism spectrum disorder that is characterized by impaired social interaction, by repetitive patterns of behaviour and restricted interests, by normal language and cognitive development but poor conversational skills and difficulty with nonverbal communication, and often by above average performance in a narrow field against a general background of impaired functioning.'

Merriam-Webster Dictionary

'My brain goes so fast; my mouth cannot keep up. My brain has a continuous dialogue going. I am working out all sorts of things all the time, there is never a gap, even when I am meant to be sleeping.

I love thinking.'

Virginia Sta Maria

CONTENTS

ASPIRATIONS

1

VERY IMPORTANT STUFF

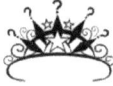

- Asperger's
- The Brain
- The Bad Pages
- I Choose
- Hyperthymesia
- Salty
- Too Much Information
- Psychologists

Asperger's

- Asperger's Syndrome was once a sub-category of Pervasive Developmental Disorder (PDD) along with Autistic Disorder and Pervasive Developmental Disorder-Not Otherwise Specified.
- Since 2013, the official diagnostic criteria for PDD changed, i.e., all the sub-categories were replaced by one single diagnostic term – Autism Spectrum Disorder (ASD). The term Asperger's Syndrome is no longer used.

- How I see Asperger's:
- Asperger's is in my family - my dad, my brother, my son Aaron, and me.
- I operate from a logical intelligence. My ways can look weird, but doing what others do is not logical to me.
- I need to learn social skills; they don't come naturally. Socialising is work for me.
- I watch people and learn but I make my own decisions about what to do. I don't live by social norms and don't follow others'.
- I need lots of time out because the outside world is so unpredictable, confusing, and therefore tiring.
- I can be childlike, naïve, and trusting.
- I have special skills: memory, singing, psychic abilities.
- I live by black and white, love and hate, strong comparisons.
- I have a great sense of humour.
- I have amazing organising skills and love things to be in order.
- I don't like change; I like life to be predictable.
- I am emotional and super aware. I use my emotions fully.
- Aspergians' brains are wired up to be more aware and sensitive to our surroundings. All my senses are heightened.

The Brain

- My way of looking at the brain is that an artistic person has more electrical impulses (wires) going into the right side of the brain and a logical person has more wires going into the left side of the brain.
- If an artistic person wants to be better at maths, they can learn, they just place the numbers into a visual pattern. When you practice the visual pattern over and over you then make new wires into the maths (left) side of the brain.
- The same is for the front/social part of the brain. Aspergian people need to learn social lessons and then there will be more wires made into the front of the brain.
- Once you learn a process, practice it and practice it, and make those wires.
- Aspies can learn to socialise with a logical brain, not a social brain.

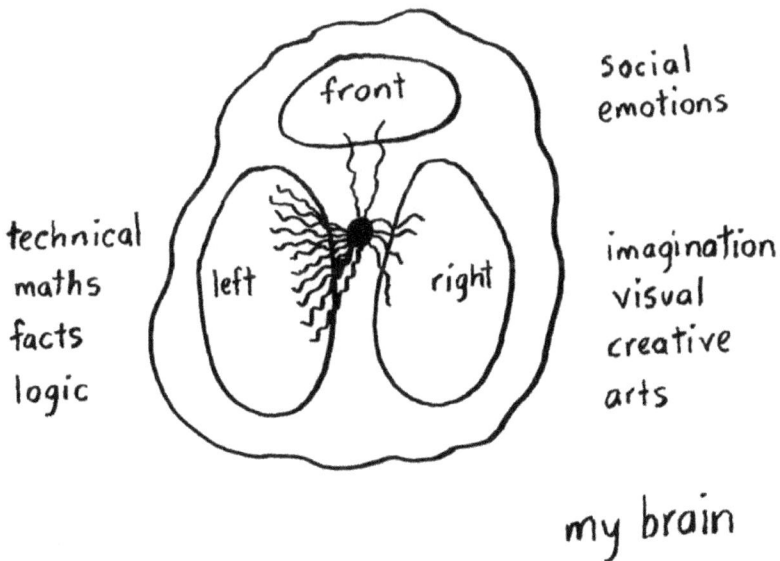

front

social
emotions

technical
maths
facts
logic

left

right

imagination
visual
creative
arts

my brain

The Bad Pages

I will keep the bad news to these few pages. They don't have any boxes or bullet points. I like to keep the boxes and bullet points for the good pages.

Dad — my father was born in England and placed into an orphanage at birth. He was shipped to Australia at the age of seven when Britain was still sending orphans overseas. He was placed into an Australian orphanage.

Mum — during the war, my mother was placed into an orphanage as a toddler in Holland.

I was born in Perth, Western Australia in 1965. I have three brothers, one older and two younger.

My childhood was not easy.

Neglect:

I was not taught basic life skills e.g., showering, even though I wet my bed for seventeen years (stress) and then slept in the same piss sheets every night. I was not taught to brush my hair or teeth, wear shoes or use cutlery. In Year One of school (age 5/6), everyone had to stand up, military style, and have our hair, nails, face and odour checked. If you were clean, you could sit down. I never got to sit down. My early school reports stated 'Virginia is aggressive and stinks'.

When I left home at nineteen, there were many basic life skills that I didn't know. Aspergians need to be shown how.

Physical Abuse:

There was always violence in my house. Beatings were random. If my dad was in a bad mood or hurt himself, someone would be beaten. The bashings became really bad after my youngest brother was born. He was born with black hair, so my dad came to the conclusion that he was not his child (my father's first kids were born with blonde hair).

My brother was bashed unconscious three times and was always covered in multi-coloured bruises from old to new. One of my 'Aspie skills', my super hearing, meant that I could hear my dad coming home on his motorbike. It gave me, my brothers (and the dog) time to scatter like mice to our rooms until we knew what mood he was in.

Mental Abuse:

My dad never called me 'Virginia'. His favourite name for me was 'Hairy

Maggot'. I also got 'bitch', 'mole', 'she', and 'Gina' (see the Gina story later in the book to see how this affected me later in life).

Sexual Abuse:

When I was seven years old, I was sexually abused by a person from my dad's orphanage. The police were involved, but no further action was taken because it was advised that I wouldn't cope well in court. One night we were coming home, and the abuser was at our front door. Dad drove past our house. I asked why we didn't stop, and Dad said, 'If I meet him, I will chop him up with an axe and kill him.' As an Aspergian, I take things literally, so this really disturbed me. It made me feel fearful and confused. I was worried about the man, wondering why my dad wanted to hurt him - the man hurt me, not my dad.

Another time was when I was ten years old. I followed some girls from school, with a boy who was a few years older than us. He asked us if we had our periods yet. Then he took us one by one into the bushes. I was last.

He made me lie down with my pants off and he lay on top of me. There was no penetration. I wasn't really scared, because the other girls had come back OK, and he paid us. I never got pocket money at home, so I wanted the money.

All through childhood and my adult life I was scared of old men (because of the abuse at age 7) and would hide whenever I saw one. I also had issues when changing my son Aaron's nappies for the first few months because I felt I was abusing him. I had to work hard to change my brain, to learn that I was helping him, doing good and not bad.

Car Accident:

When I was five years old, I was riding my bike on the road and a car headed straight for me and ran me over. I spent six weeks in hospital. A few years later, I was in the post office with Mum, and we saw the guy who had hit me.

Mum said to me, 'That is the guy who ran you over, I want to run him over.' I looked at the man; he seemed old and feeble. Again, I was confused why my mum would want to hurt him. Both my parents had disturbing, distorted views of revenge.

I have blocked the car accident itself from my memory, but my subconscious remembers, and I am still jumpy around roads.

Crime:

I was forced to go into shops and steal, mainly clothes. I would have to put on new clothes in the shop, go back to the car, change out of the new clothes, and then go back into the shop for more. I didn't want to, it was very stressful.

My parents would also go on late-night building site raids and take all of us kids with them. I was usually asleep when they put me in the car but would wake up as bricks and other items were loaded in and around me. Our barbeque area and enormous back shed were built entirely from stolen items.

Socialising:

I can only remember people visiting our house around four times. Dad would insult them, and they wouldn't return. Both my parents were orphans so there were no aunts, uncles or cousins, just us six.

The Dogs:

We never kept any particular dog for very long. Dad would dump them when they dug holes. I don't know why we kept getting more dogs, it baffles me. Now that I have a family of my own, we look after our dogs and keep them all their lives, they are not disposable.

Mum:

When I was almost three years old, my mum gave birth to a still-born baby and also had a horrific horse and cart accident. She spent three months in hospital, and I spent those months in a children's home. In 1968 still-born babies were just taken from the mother and then a whole lot of babies' bodies were put in the same hole at the cemetery with no headstone. Mothers were told to go home and forget about it. There was no counselling or medication. My mum was always depressed and in a daze.

Naïve:

When I moved out of home at nineteen years of age, three things happened that show how naive I was about the evils in the world:

1. I lived in a complex of eight units. My friend lived across the road from me. One day I went over to visit her, but she was not at home. Her flatmate was there, and he followed me back to my place, wanting to know where I lived. He came into my unit and asked where my bedroom was. I showed him. He threw me on the bed and started to strangle me. He was wearing black leather gloves, and his stare was intense. I struggled and his face changed; he got up and walked out. I just thought that it was all some kind of joke.

2. I was at a beer garden with my flatmate's friend (FF). I was laughing with some guys when one guy picked me up and threw me over his shoulder. Then he and his friend ran out to the carpark to his car. FF was yelling at him to put

me down. He threw me into the back of his car and his friend got into the driver's seat. FF was screaming hysterically, and the guy let me go. Again, I thought it was his way of joking.

3. When I was twenty-one years old, I was raped. I offered to accompany a friend's visiting mates out to dinner (the friend was away; I was just being nice).

It turned out that one of the mates was a serial rapist. He encouraged me to compete with him in drinking shots, until I was so drunk I could barely walk. He said he would drive me home. His mate looked concerned, but he did not stop his friend or try to help me. The drive home included a detour and sexual assault. He later bragged about his conquest, another one of his 'scores'.

In all three cases, each of the guys had premeditated his actions. I didn't go to the police, especially with the rape because I am just like other girls who are sexually assaulted and believe it was their fault.

I still feel very used and embarrassed about it. I have decided not to take action; having hyperthymesia (excessive memory), means I don't just recall the past, I re-live it in full detail.

I met Oliver when I was 22 years old and without knowing it, he kept me safe. I did not put myself into bad situations because I would say 'I can't do that; I have a boyfriend.'

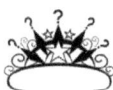

I Choose

- I wrote the Bad Pages to show that:
- I have chosen not to let my dysfunctional family background define the family I have now. I think of it as changing my ancestry. So many people just copy the same behaviour, never changing, generation after generation, just continued crap. I learned what not to do.
- Oliver and I never hit our son, Aaron. He was loved unconditionally. We taught him hygiene skills and showed him how to be a good person. He only knows how to be in a safe, loving home. We have created a new, positive family template that he can use when he decides to start his own family.
- I have achieved more than anyone I know. My childhood did not hinder me.
- I spent a lot of time with psychologists. Abused children and Aspergians have much in common: high anxiety, senses over-heightened, no friends, emotionally unstable, craving stability and security. For years and years, I was diagnosed as being from an abused childhood and not as an Aspergian. It was through my adult counselling with Winnie that my ongoing issues were identified as Asperger's symptoms rather than just the result of abuse.
- I am always thinking and working on myself. As Winnie told me once, I have a 'matter of fact' way of thinking which has protected me. I now think about my past from a technical view and how I can work through things. Being identified with a traumatic childhood means I am a victim. But being diagnosed with Asperger's is powerful for me. I love being Aspergian and unique.
- Since meeting Oliver and having a child together, I now have a family that has helped me work through the Bad Things.

Hyperthymesia

- Hyperthymesia means 'excessive memory'.

- I always thought everyone remembered everything, like me. I thought people were lying when they said they didn't remember.

- My earliest memories are from when I was two years old. I remember the house I lived in, my bedroom and the backyard. I also remember the time I spent in Ngala Children's Home where I was sent while my mother was recovering from her accident.

- When I remember, I also re-live. I am there and I can look around the scene. All my senses are involved - I can see, hear, smell, taste and feel all the details.

- I can also pick up objects and go back in my mind to where I got them and look around the shop.

- My memory was not useful in school. I couldn't remember stuff for exams. I just randomly remember general information. This is a typical trait for someone with hyperthymesia - it is not like having perfect memory.

- I amaze myself with the knowledge or jokes that come from me. I don't know where the information comes from. It is like a Google search.

- If I remember something, I will remember all other common information. One thought will trigger another and another. I have no control over it.

- Before I learned about hyperthymesia, one event stuck in my mind. Oliver and I had placed realistic-looking fake butterflies on the family room walls. Oliver said he didn't want them there anymore, so we took them down and stored them. Three years later, I wanted to put them up again. I believed Oliver would remember, like I did, and that he wouldn't want them back up on the walls. Of course, he couldn't remember, and he now said he liked them there.

Salty

- Age: 11 years
- Because of my hyperthymesia, when I remember something, it triggers all the other details to come to me. I re-live and re-feel the whole day.
- For example, I remember the first time I had takeaway food in January 1977.
- My family had travelled to Sydney, and we were staying in a caravan park.
- Mum and dad had run out of money, and they were trying to organise a loan from my dad's boss. They told me and my brothers to stay in the caravan park.
- We played in the shower block with another kid.
- When my parents came back it was late, so they gave us takeaway food for dinner.
- The tub of potato and gravy was very salty and whenever I remember it my mouth will start watering.
- I re-live and re-feel that whole day - the games we played in the shower block, the trip from the takeaway shop back to the caravan park, eating my potato and gravy on the fold-down seat of our panel van, and using my logic to give my dad directions when we got lost on the way back (neither parent gave me any praise for solving the problem, just silence).
- This is a feature of hyperthymesia, one recall triggers many others associated with it, it is not controllable.

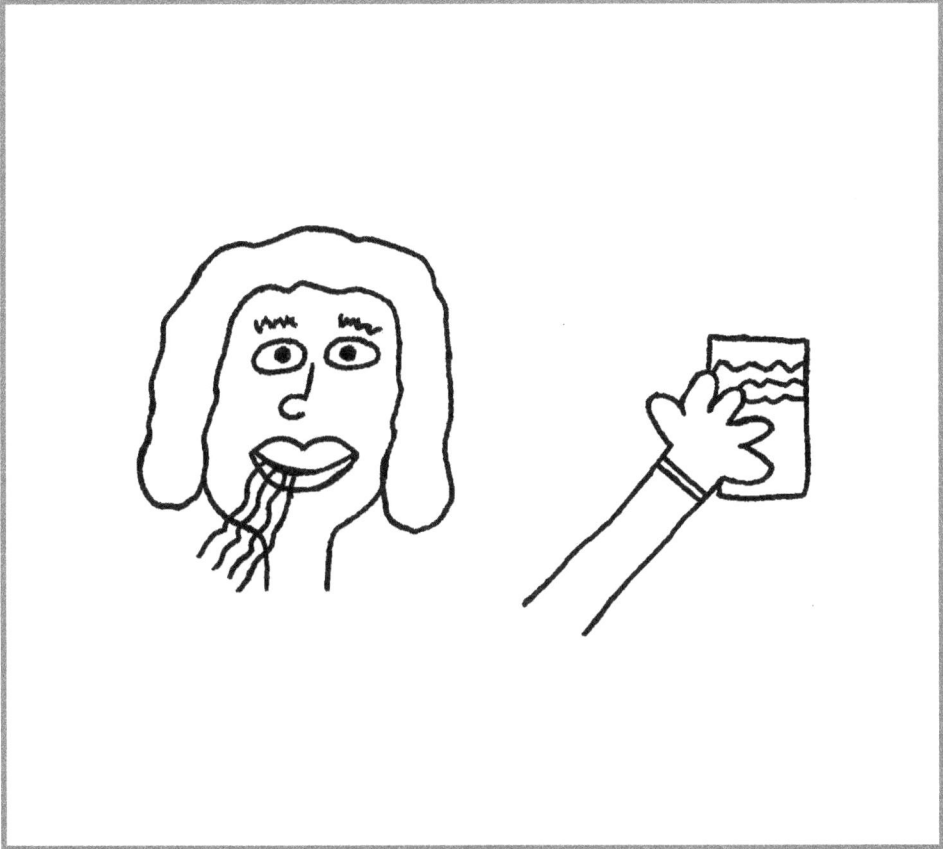

Too Much Information

- I am often asked if my constant thinking and memory are tiring - no, I love them.
- One day on the way home in the car, I told Oliver all the things I remembered on this one road. He asked me to be quiet, he couldn't handle that much information.

saw Fatal Attraction movie here 1987 X

X went to a party down this road - mid 1980s

hired trailer from here in 2009   X

X Mary worked in bank here - late 1990s

bought car here in 1988   X

the cafe here sold that delicious X sausage roll

Waffle Way

X bought kitchen tiles from here in 2006

X bought shelves from here - early 2000s

X bought our treadmill here in 2007

X Kevin had that accident here and had to go to hospital - 2002

X Stuart worked here - he married Kate in 1991

X our dog went here for that operation in 1995

✳ Note: I did drive down a road and tell Oliver all the things I remembered but this page is as an example only. ✳

Psychologists

- My first experience of psychologists was when I was diagnosed with depression in 1996. I was thirty years old. My dog had to be put down and my friend's dad, who had been my 'substitute dad', died in the same week.

- It started my time with psychologists (seven in total over twenty years) and the same question they all ask is, 'Tell me about your childhood.'

- I have found this doesn't work for me because I don't just remember, I re-live my childhood. It seems that neurotypical people love to just talk, and it helps them. It doesn't help me, it just takes me straight back into the trauma.

- I kept going to psychologists because I felt my mind just wasn't right. I was so confused with the world.

- In 2014, at the age of forty-nine, I was finally diagnosed with Asperger's by clinical psychologist Dr. Winnie Yu Pow Blake.

- Winnie knows all about Asperger's and speaks Aspie language. She knows I love lists, stories and formulas and all her solutions are based around that. The therapy is more sterile, working with information rather than just talking and venting.

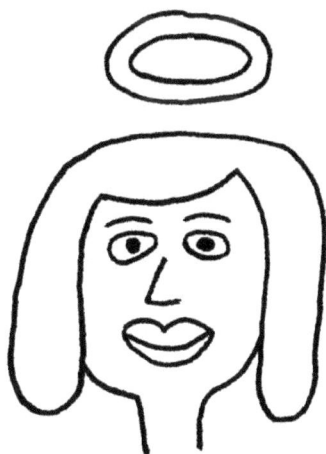

Winnie

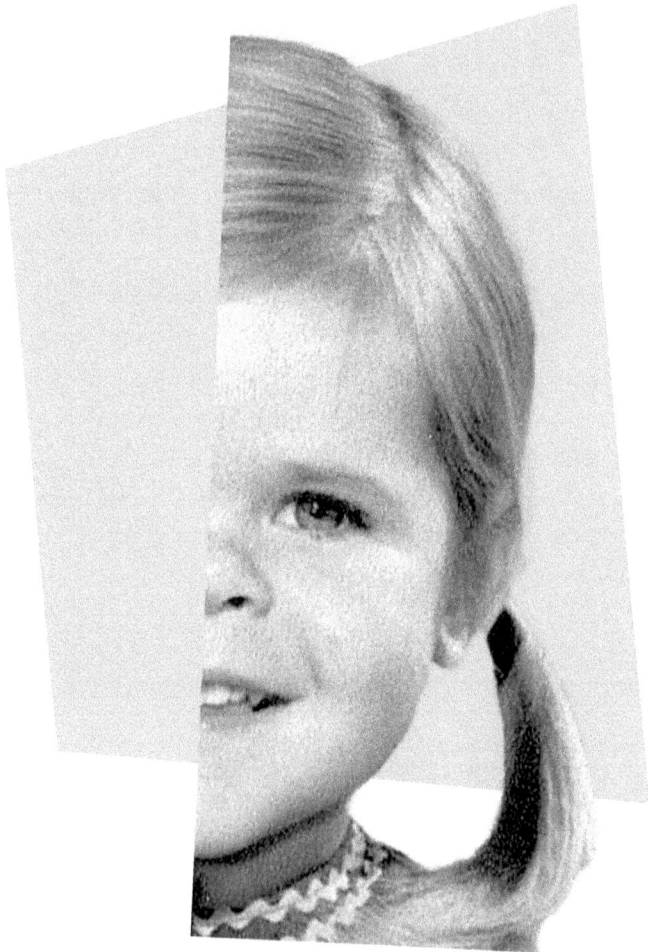

2

EARLY DAYS

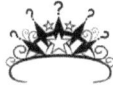

- School Life
- Brownies
- Game On
- Tell Me More
- Name Calling
- First Friend
- First Boyfriend
- Perfect Flatmate
- Perfect Match

School Life

- I never went to any sleepovers or birthday parties.
- In primary school, I would line up toys on the oval and wait for 'friends' to come.
- I would beat other kids up. My thinking was that the boys would let me hang out with them if they saw I was tough.
- I spent my lunch time in the library or walking around the oval.
- In my school life, I had sporadic friends at times.
- I was OK at maths and science but didn't understand English at all, too much guessing for me.
- I loved to do stats of the kids in my class, their names and where they sat. At home I would put the information into a map.
- I didn't understand gossip, bitching, teasing or manipulating but I could see the other students doing it.

* Note : example only

Mrs Lesson

me	Mary	Bruce	Nick	Kevin
Anna	Tina	Sarah	Tom	Harry
Cindy	Liam	Sam	Neil	Karen
Emily	Kate	Greg	Chris	Henry

Brownies

- When I was eight years old, I was in Brownies (Girl Guides).
- I loved it, all the rules and routines and art and craft.
- On one occasion we went on a camp to a country town. I was billeted to a couple's house with three other Brownies.
- The other girls would go out somewhere, but I stayed at the house with the couple, watching TV. I sat on the floor between the lady's legs (she was in an armchair). She brushed my hair with a very soft hairbrush. I had never experienced this type of attention before.
- My parents did not tell the Brownie group leaders about my bed wetting. At night, of course, I wet the bed. I was devastated.
- In the morning, the other girls did not make their beds, but I did because I wanted to hide the fact that my bed was wet. I wanted the woman of the house to think I was a good person.
- Once I was back at home, I refused to go to Brownies anymore because I truly believed the couple would be angry and call the police and the police would arrest me.
- I still have my Brownie badge and book.

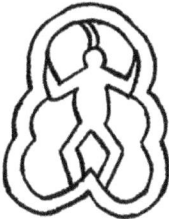

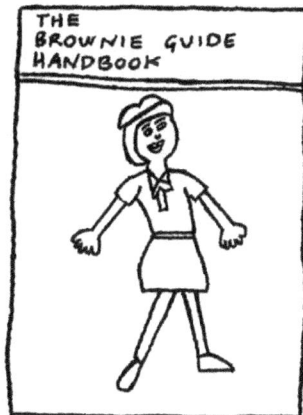

Game On

- Age: teens
- At school, I was no good at sports.
- For some reason the ball always ended up in my face.
- When teams were picked, I was not last. I beat the girl with one arm and the girl who rocked from side to side.
- I felt that the sports teacher liked me. Once when my class was playing netball, I just ran up and down the court, the girls avoiding me. The ball went out of court near me. I bent down and picked up the ball and a girl rushed over and snatched it from my hands. The teacher yelled 'Just let her touch the bloody ball!'
- I got to throw the ball back into the game.

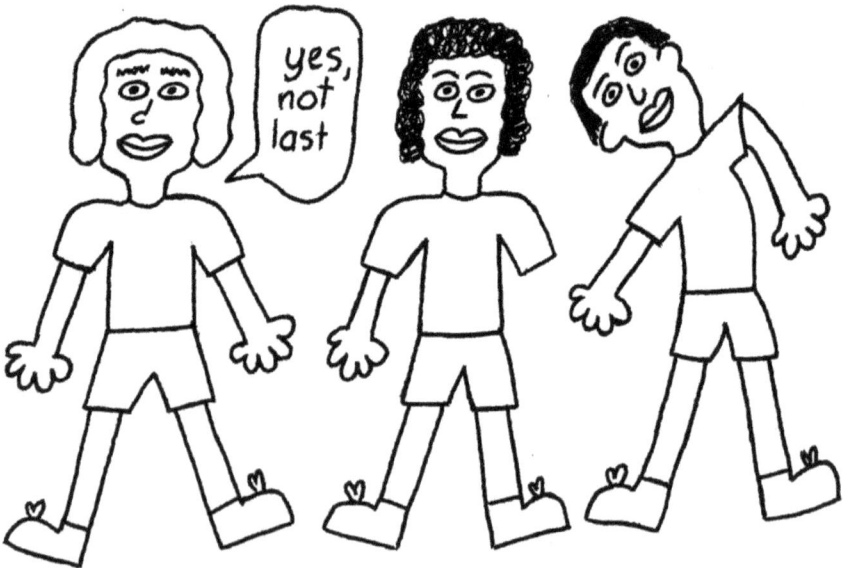

Tell Me More

- Age: teens
- In high school, the big movie at the time was *Grease* with the actors Olivia Newton John and John Travolta.
- I rarely went to movies and then only with mum.
- Some girls in my class were standing around, talking very excitedly about seeing the movie together on the weekend.
- I stood close enough to listen but not be noticed.
- I just could not understand how they organised it, how they met on the weekend, how they paid, all the details, like a small child wonders how their teacher does normal things outside of school.

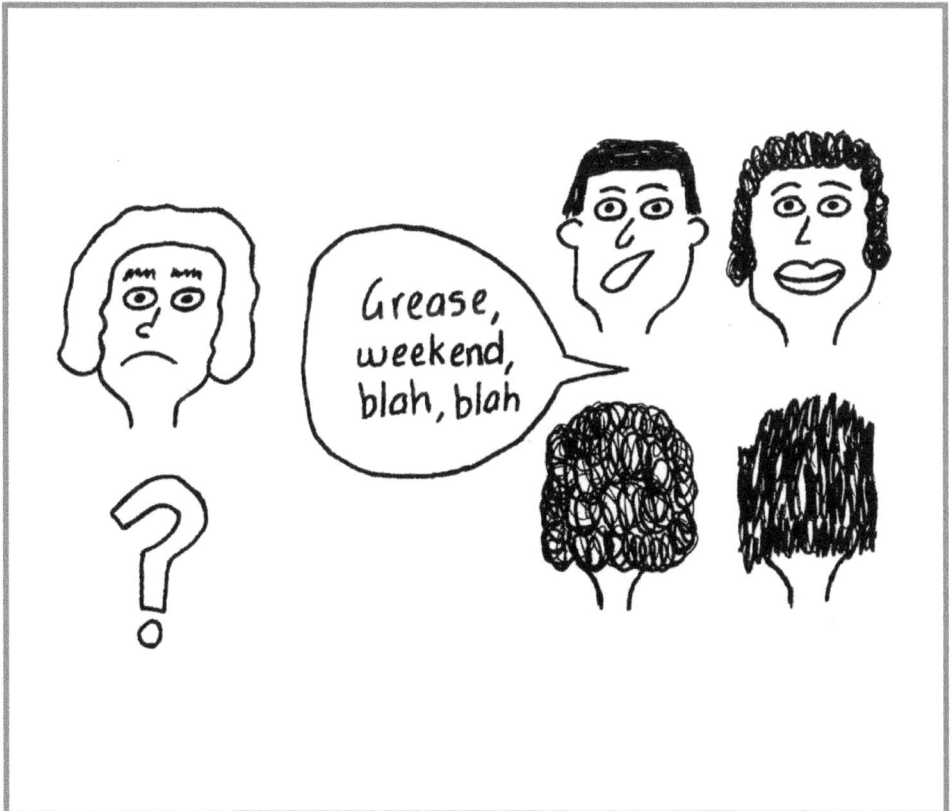

Name Calling

- Age: teens
- At high school, we learned about body parts and there were some clever responses.
- As I walked around, some students would yell out to me, 'Hey, Vagina, where's your boyfriend Penis?' I thought this was so funny and would laugh, so after a while the name calling stopped. I think bullies don't like to be laughed at.
- Another situation was with a group of girls who always asked me, 'Are you still wearing a rag?' I thought they were referring to my clothing, because I always wore second-hand clothes. I answered them 'Yes' and laughed.

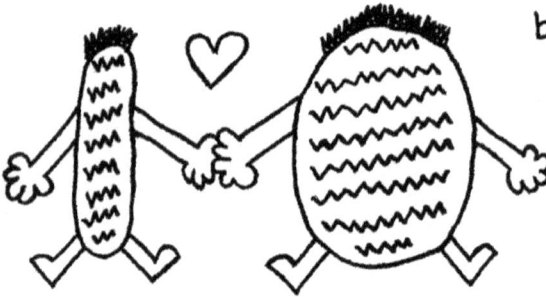

boyfriend and girlfriend

blurred for your 'Pupil Protection'

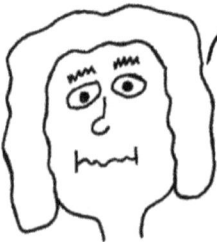

Thinking Back...
'On the rag' is slang for having your period and wearing a pad.

First Friend

- At the age of seventeen, Mum took me to the Technical and Further Education (TAFE) college in the city to choose a course. I chose Accounting Machine Practice because of the maths and machine operating. This was in the days before computers. I didn't know anything about working in an office and had no thoughts about the future.

- I met my first true friend at the TAFE college. We discovered that we had both been born in the same hospital, twelve hours apart, in the same ward.

- With 'First Friend' I went to my first-ever sleepovers and family parties.

- Her parents could tell I had had an abused childhood. I would stand against walls and watch everyone, ready to protect myself. I would jump if anyone came near me.

- These people became something of a family for me, and I came to think of her dad as my substitute father.

- 'First Friend' was a very touchy-touchy person. I didn't get affection as an older child/teenager, and so her touching me made me feel very confused. I liked her being affectionate to me, but I liked boys, not girls. I didn't understand about non-sexual affection.

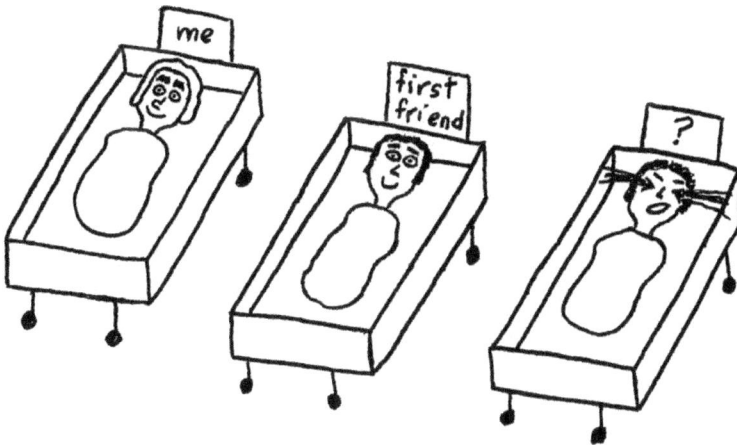

First Boyfriend

- Age: late teens
- I met at my friend's boyfriend's house. We were all going to a house party.
- I was to travel in the boyfriend's friend's car. I had never met him before.
- On the way to the party, at some traffic lights, he takes his penis out and rests it in his lap, points down and asks me, 'Hey, what do you think about this?'
- I looked and then did my usual answer – shoulder shrug and 'I don't know.'
- So, I'm thinking he wants to be my boyfriend. I'd never had a boyfriend before and I always thought there were a few more steps such as 'What is your name?', 'Where do you live?', 'Do you like cats or dogs?', and 'Would you like to go for a coffee?' But maybe that was just in the movies.
- When we arrived at the party, he ran off and left me at the car.
- I followed him inside the house and out to the backyard. I tried to catch up with him to discuss which movie we were going to see on our first date.
- He kept moving away when he saw me. I kept pursuing.
- Eventually he hid from me, and I couldn't find him, so I went and found my friend.

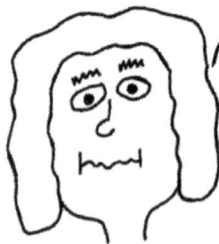

Thinking Back...

I didn't understand, the whole thing really confused me. I really thought he wanted to be my boyfriend. I now realise he was probably embarrassed, and my response was not what he expected. Other girls would either have rooted* him or screamed at him.

* 'root' is an Australian slang word for 'having sex'

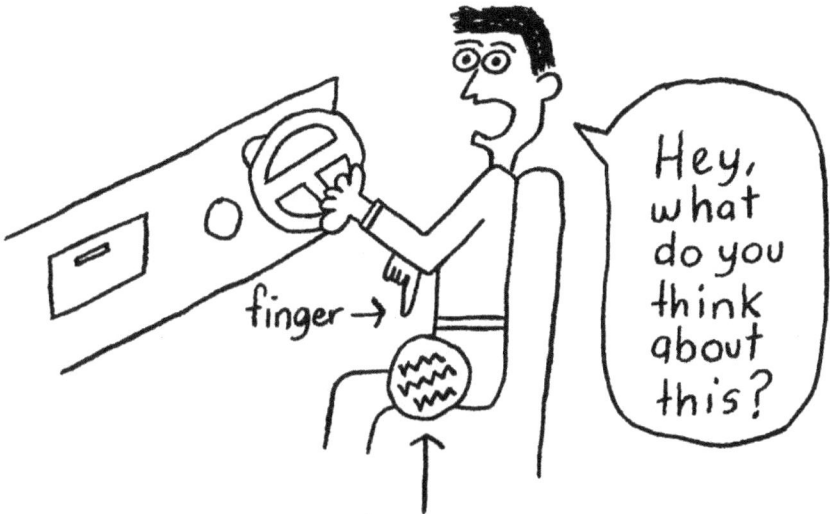

Perfect Flatmate

- Age: 19
- My mum had made dad leave two years before, but things were still difficult at home.
- I got a job. A girl at work asked me to share a house with her, so I moved out.
- I was the perfect flatmate. I was so naïve - I didn't smoke, drink or do drugs, was quiet and very willing to take advice from others because I simply had no idea how to do most things and wanted to learn.
- I watched my flatmate showering (not actually watching her have a shower, just taking note of her routine), brushing her teeth, her breakfast habits, how she used cutlery, what clothes she chose to wear. I just watched and copied everything she did.
- I was introduced to parties, going to the movies, boys, alcohol, clothes, make-up, shopping, hanging out with a group of friends, how to socialise, nightclubs and pubs.
- I was like an excited puppy, wanting to learn and soak up everything.
- Note: I was having daily showers, but I still stank. Eventually I worked out that I had to wash my towel. I didn't know this. I figured it out when the towel became really, really smelly.

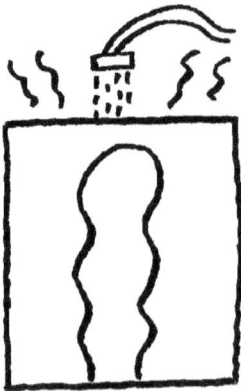

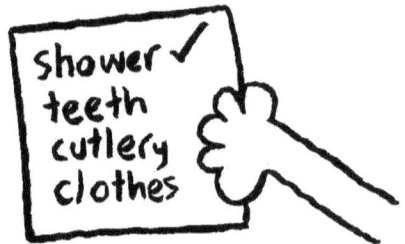

24

Perfect Match

- Age: 22
- My 'First Friend' moved into a new shared flat with a man named Oliver.
- I used to visit her and then I saw Oliver and I would visit even if she wasn't there.
- Oliver and I noticed each other, and we both used my friend as a go-between, asking her 'What does she/he think about me?'
- In the end she told us to leave her alone and just go out with each other.
- Oliver had an astrology book and I checked out our compatibility. It was good except it said, 'Keep him entertained or he will wander.' I have definitely entertained him with my Aspie ways and humour. He says I entertain him too much.
- An interesting thing about our relationship is we fit all the criteria to make an Aspie/neurotypical relationship work e.g., age gap (Oliver is sixteen years older than me), Oliver was in a caring profession (training to be a psychiatric nurse) and we are both from different cultures.
- Oliver is from a Eurasian background. Neither of us knew about my Asperger's. So, when I over-reacted, I was just being 'Australian'.

Flatmate Required

I am very handsome and require a female flatmate who has a beautiful friend
Phone Oliver
9123 4567

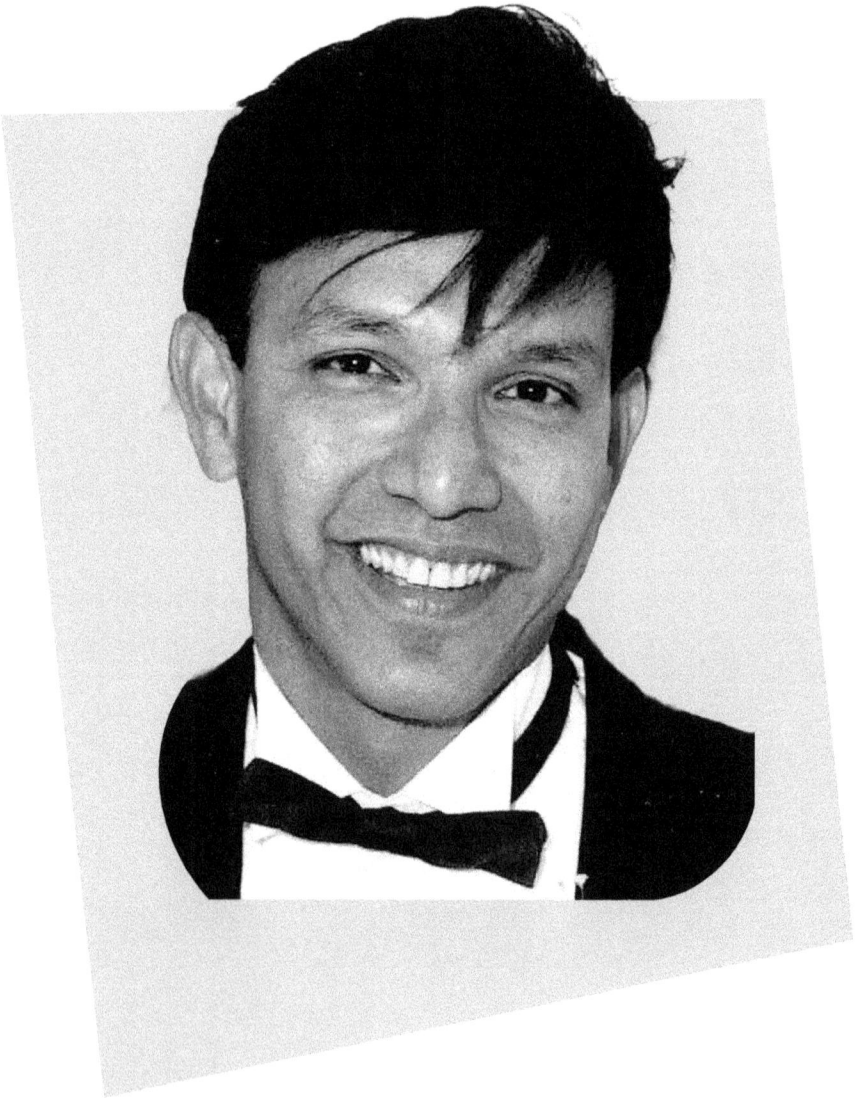

3

FAMILY

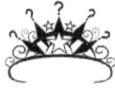

- Oliver
- Dating Skills
- Still Waiting
- Oliver's Parents
- Visiting Doctors
- Pregnant

Oliver

- Extra extreme handsome (see scale below)
- Intelligent. I like that we both can talk smart talk.
- He is not overly social and doesn't do Facebook.
- He is confident and independent.
- Oliver accepted me unconditionally and gave me the stability I craved.
- We both love the bush but not the beach.
- We both love learning.
- Oliver became my 'Special Interest'. I was obsessed with him 100%.
- Oliver loves having fun and laughed at my Aspie humour. He loved my innocence and me being different.
- He taught me social rules such as not to do 'double dipping' (e.g., when you dip a snack into the dipping sauce at a party, take a bite, then dip the bitten part back in the sauce).
- At social events, he would walk in first so I could follow and copy him.
- In our business, he attends to the emails and talking to people. I do the accounts, tax and organising.

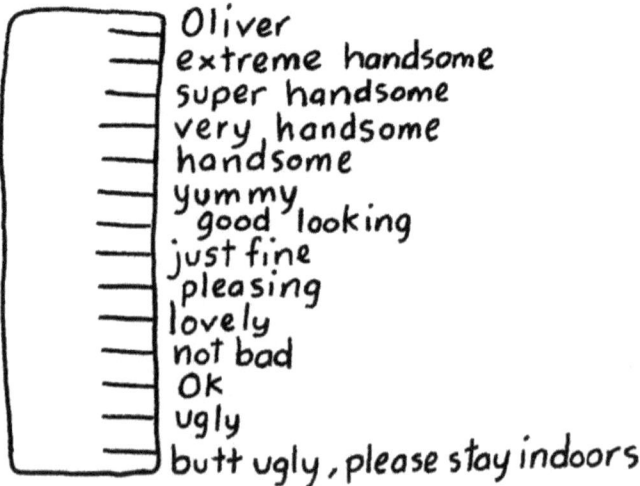

Oliver
extreme handsome
super handsome
very handsome
handsome
yummy
good looking
just fine
pleasing
lovely
not bad
Ok
ugly
butt ugly, please stay indoors

Dating Skills

- Age: early 20s
- On our second date, Oliver took me to see the movie *Crocodile Dundee II* starring the actors Paul Hogan as Mick and Linda Kowalski as Sue.
- In the movie, the character Sue takes off her bra without removing her top. The character Mick reacts in shock. How was she able to perform such an amazing feat?
- I thought, 'I can do that,' so I very carefully removed my bra without Oliver noticing anything.
- When we were back outside, I handed him my bra.

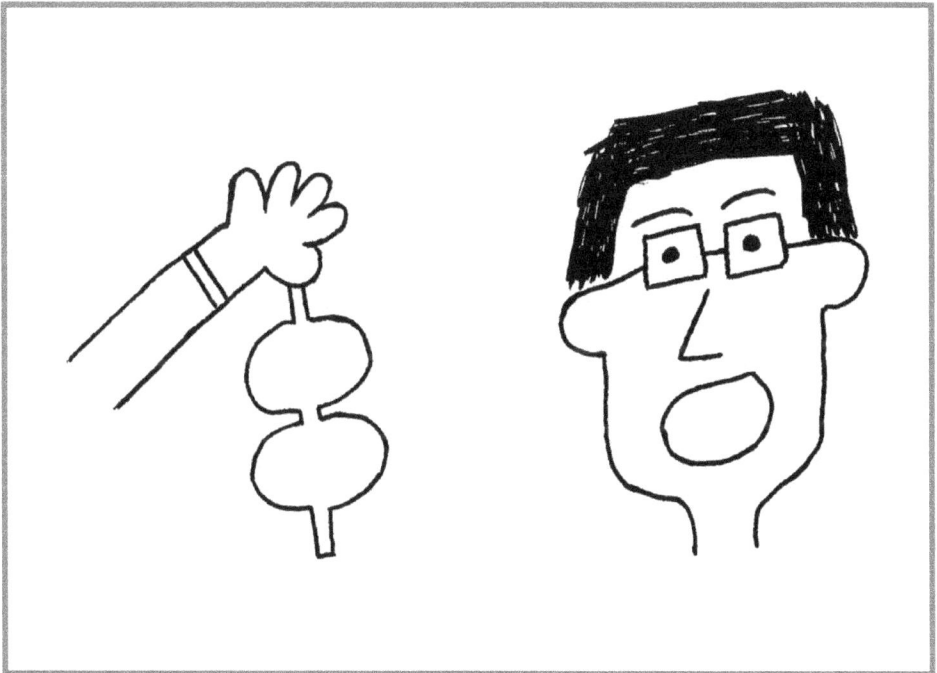

- Note: during the movie, I dropped a chocolate-covered peanut. I bent down and picked it up and put it in my mouth. It was a chocolate-covered sultana. Mmmm yum, how long had that been there?

Still Waiting

- Age: early 20s
- I had a few boyfriends before Oliver. They would say things to me like 'When we go out, please behave', 'Stop acting so immature, grow up' and 'Why are you doing that, that way?'
- All the relationships seem to end around the two-month mark.
- I had been dating Oliver around two months.
- We were living with another couple in a tiny two-bedroom unit.
- One day Oliver said, 'Let's go for a walk.' I thought, 'Oh, here we go, break-up time.'
- We walked around the streets, and I was very quiet, just waiting for the bad news. We arrived back home and Oliver hadn't said anything, he didn't break up with me.
- At home, I thought he was still going to break up with me, he just couldn't do it on the walk.
- I was in tension for days.
- We have been together for thirty-six years.

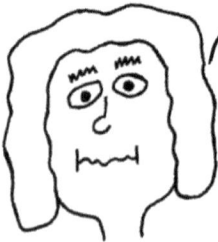

Thinking Back...
All the other relationships ended because I wasn't acting like other girls. Oliver loved me because I wasn't like other girls.

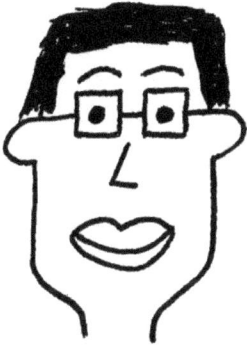

Oliver's Parents

- I remember the first time I met Oliver's parents. His dad was quiet, but his mum was very friendly and wanted me to sit and eat.
- Over the years I have learned they are the parents everyone dreams of having.
- Oliver's parents showed me how parents should be.
- Their house was always so positive and secure. There were never any 'mind games' such as guilt, shaming or manipulation. I felt a calmness and steadiness and never any erratic emotions. I always felt safe and welcome.
- When we were starting our financial journey, Oliver's dad believed in us and helped us by loaning us money for our first big venture.
- Both his parents were so proud of us and never jealous. They wanted to know what we were up to and gave us lots of help.
- We knew they loved and supported us unconditionally.

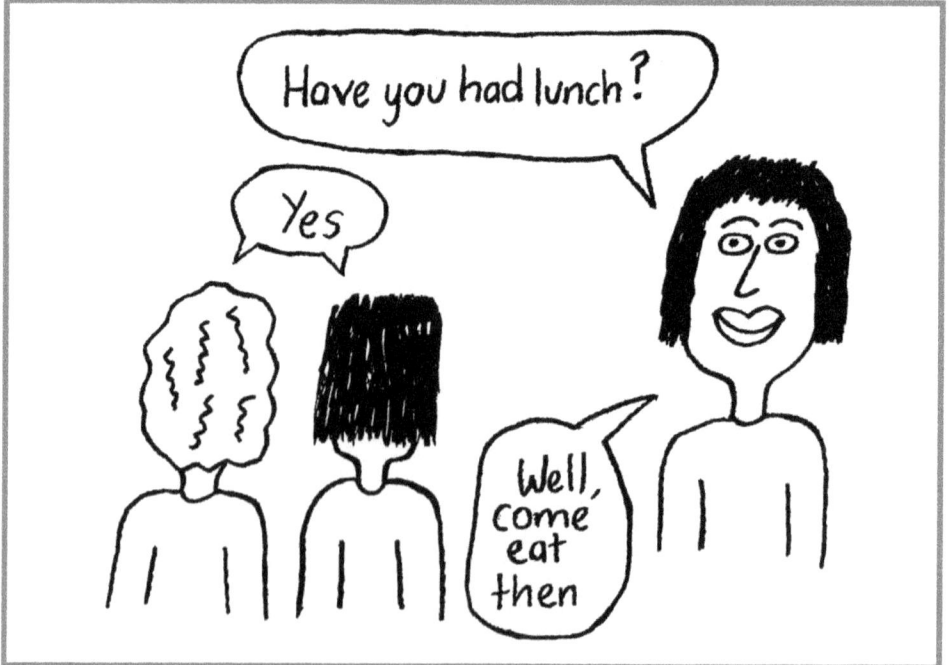

Visiting Doctors

- Age: late 20s
- Our son is an IVF baby.
- During the embryo transfer, my doctor asked me if it would be alright if five visiting doctors could watch. I was used to opening my legs during all the fertility treatments, so I agreed - having more people looking was fine with me.
- I was lucky the embryo transfer took place before phone cameras were a thing, because these days, the tourists (doctors) would probably want to take selfies with my 'Quokka' (a small, hairy marsupial found on Perth's Rottnest Island).

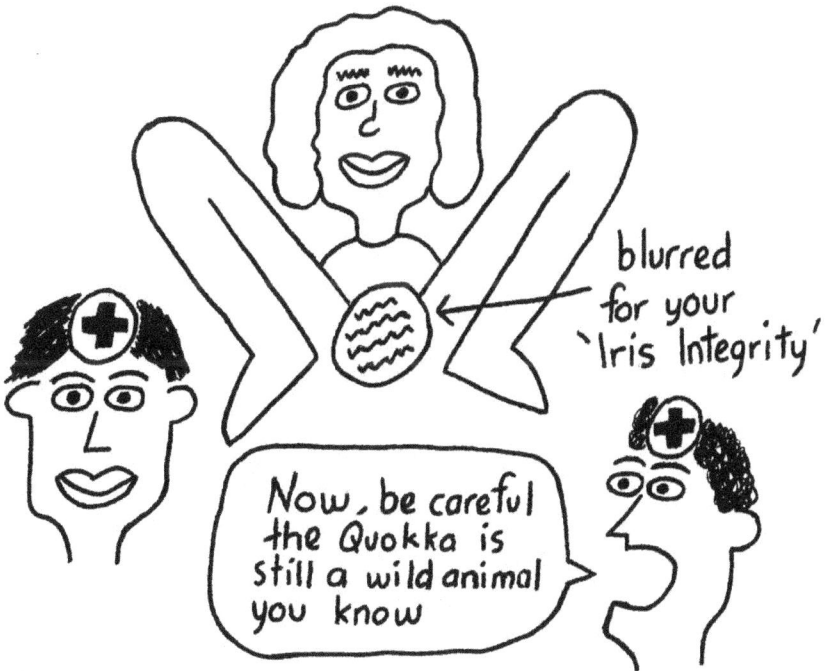

Pregnant

- Oliver and I wanted so much to have a baby together, but both of us had fertility issues.

- After many interventions, we tried IVF and were lucky to have Aaron after the first attempt.

- During IVF, every morning I had to have three needles: one in my arm, one in my thigh and one in my butt. The one in my butt made my leg numb which made walking interesting. I had to wear long sleeves to hide the bruises on my arm.

- In the mornings (needle time), the many waiting women would talk together. I stayed quiet, keeping to myself.

- During my pregnancy, I was not excited because I just didn't believe it. When my stomach was big, Oliver and I were crying because it had seemed so impossible – so many 'no' results.

- I didn't know that there were tests that I should have. One time Aaron (foetus) was not moving in my womb. He was usually an active baby. I was worried, so I went to the clinic. They were amazed that I had had no tests so far.

- I just didn't know to ask questions. I am blind to what is going on. Other women learn through socialising and asking questions. What questions do I ask? I was just doing my best to figure things out and follow the ways that seemed logical to me. The doctors and nurses had no idea that I didn't know to ask them questions.

- I remember watching birth videos for the first time in my life and was so upset; I couldn't do that.

- At six months pregnant, Aaron's head was under my ribcage, so the doctor told me to book in for a caesarean. I think I manifested that.

- The birth was easy because it was all controlled.

- After Aaron was born, I had extreme mood swings in the hospital where one moment I felt like Superman and then suicidal, but I stayed strong because I had my dream, a baby.

- After the birth I did not know that your period starts again very soon. I was not prepared with pads, so I used paper hand towels in my undies. The nurse was so angry with me when she found out.

- My childhood upbringing had no bearing on Aaron because Oliver and I learned new ways of doing things through our love of researching information. If we didn't know something, we found out. In true Aspie style, I did what felt right, not by social norms. For example, when breastfeeding I made sure to release any negative energy beforehand, I didn't want to feed Aaron 'negative milk'.

- After Aaron was born, I was involved in a play group, and I had other first-time mothers to watch and copy if I wanted to.

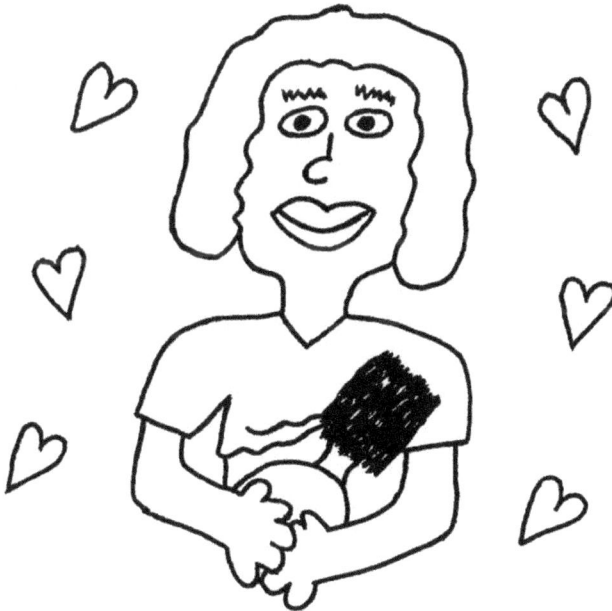

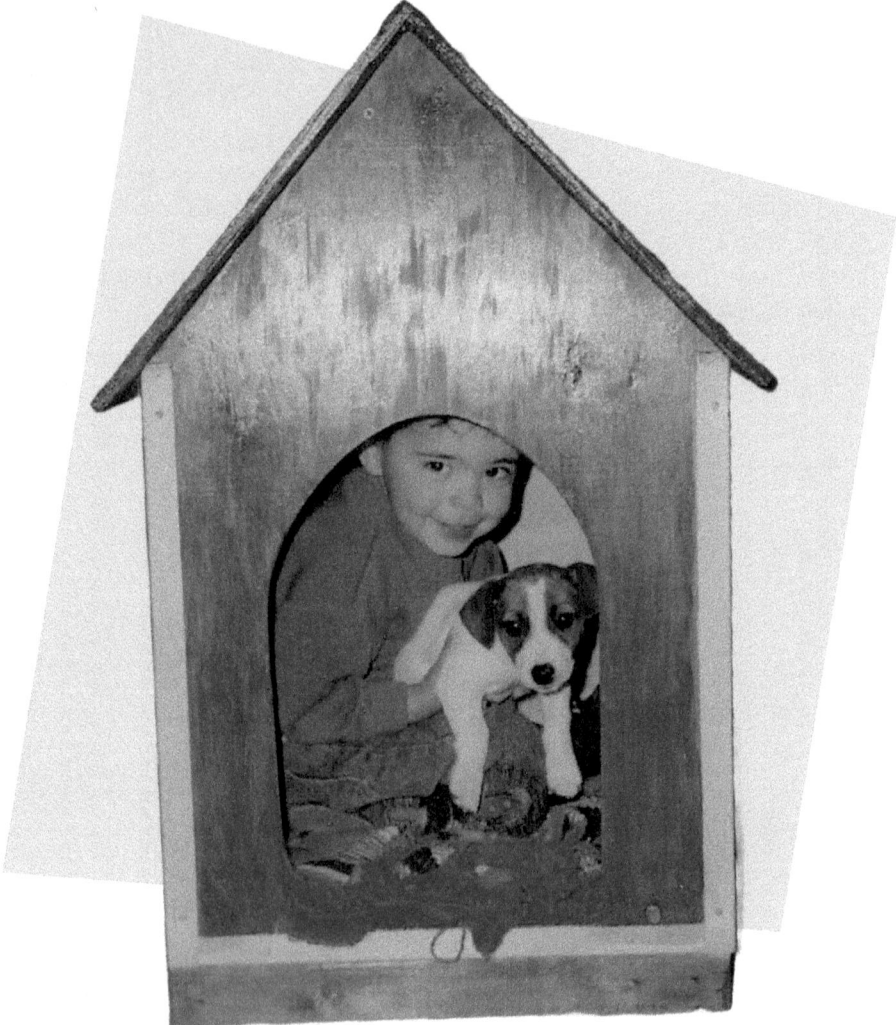

4

AARON

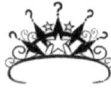

- Aaron
- No Problem
- Aaron at School
- Book Learning
- Time Wasters
- Fight
- Dreams Come True
- We Are Family

Aaron

- Aaron was a very easy child and teenager to parent.

- I parented him in a logical way, not following the norm, just what made sense to me. We did not perceive Aaron as autistic; he was not diagnosed until high school, and I was not diagnosed until later in life, so we just raised him to be himself.

- He was always so happy and busy. One moment he was in his sandpit, then playing with his dogs, next inside making something and then on his electric piano keyboard with the volume full blast.

- I loved watching him do things in his own way.

- I explained things in lots of details, how things worked and why. He loved all the information.

- When we were camping with Oliver's family, Aaron, three and a half years old, would put his toy trucks in his backpack and go to visit each of the other family members' camper trailers. He would knock on the door, and they would ask, 'Who is it?' – 'Aaron' - 'Aaron who?' Aaron would answer 'Aaron Good Boy.'

- Teaching him manners was very important to me. I remember riding my bike with Aaron when he was five. We were heading towards a bus stop full of waiting people. I yelled ahead to Aaron, 'Say excuse me!' He said 'Excuse me' and rode right through. The people moved out of the way and said 'Thank you.'

- When shopping I would let Aaron have one item he wanted. That way, he knew something in the shopping trolley was his. Over the years the number of his items grew until the conveyor belt at the checkout had one item of mine and the rest belonged to him.

- When Aaron was seven years old, I learned at a seminar to give kids an initiation when they turned thirteen. This made a lot of sense to me, so I retained this information and on Aaron's 13th birthday Oliver, Aaron and I climbed Sydney Harbour Bridge. Everyone there sang 'Happy Birthday' to him on top of the bridge.

No Problem

- Aaron always read the use-by date on food packaging. Once he found an expired jar of peanut paste. We told him it was still fine. He covered the outside of the jar with death and expiration warnings. I love his unique way of handling problems.

- Once, when Aaron was ten, we finished shopping and paid at the checkout. As we left, Aaron noticed he had some chocolate in his pocket which wasn't paid for. He started panicking. I said 'Don't worry,' and headed back to the checkout, explained and paid for the chocolate. He learned about honesty and solving problems.

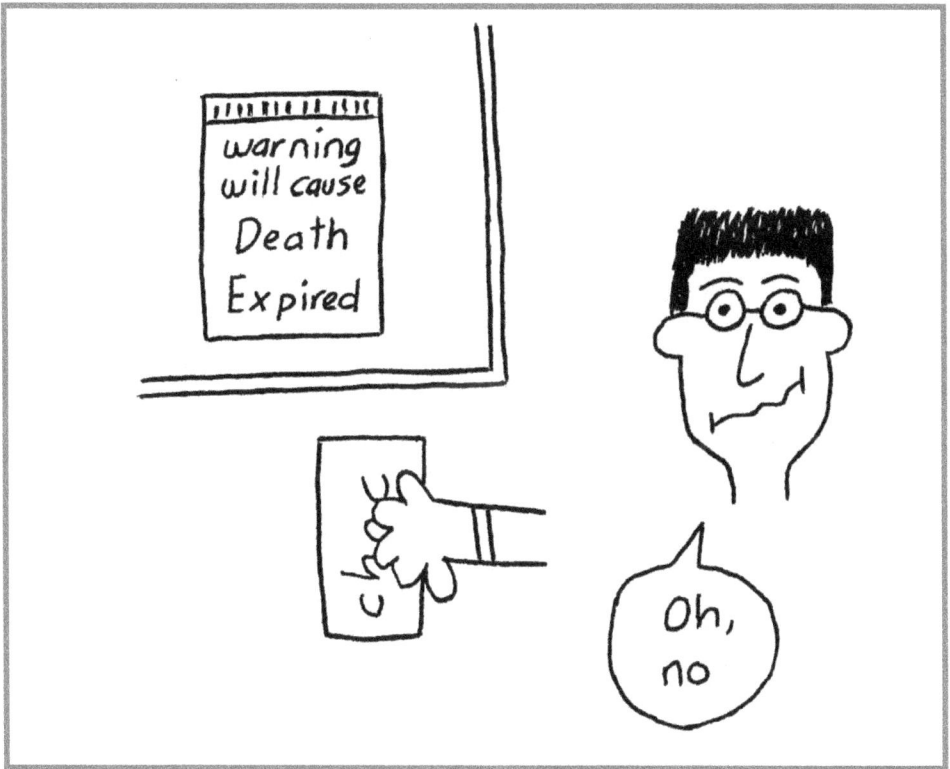

Aaron at School

- When Aaron was in Year One (5/6 years old), his teacher said Aaron was the smartest student she'd ever taught.
- In Year Two (7 years old) his teacher let him work without instructions.
- In Year Three (8 years old) when I got his first school report, he was one of the dumbest students.
- I approached the principal. Aaron was then seen by a school psychologist. The report came back that Aaron was well above average with areas of exceptional ability.
- Aaron had been bullied in Year Three by the teacher and other students so I changed him to a Montessori school on recommendation. It was an easy decision. Aaron had to be happy and free to learn at his own level.
- His Montessori class had students from Year Three to Year Seven, and a dog. This meant that Aaron could hang out with younger kids that he could more easily understand.
- During Aaron's secondary school orientation, I was told to have him assessed because they noticed how he stood out by avoiding everyone.
- Aaron was twelve years old when he was diagnosed with Asperger's.
- Once Aaron had the diagnosis, nothing happened at school - no support, only ten minutes of extra time to prepare for exams.
- If Aaron had not been diagnosed, he would have just thought secondary school was hard and tried to fit in, but because he had a label (Asperger's) he felt paranoid that he was weird.

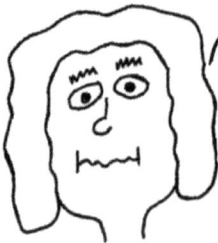

Thinking Back...
I would have let Aaron wait until adulthood to choose for himself if he wanted a diagnosis.

Book Learning

- Aaron found high school hard. It was very social. He was also super aware of his diagnosis and didn't like being different.
- He spent his lunchtime in the school library and walking the school grounds, just the way I did throughout my school days.
- The students carried their books at their sides to each class. Aaron carried his in front even though it was uncomfortable. He did this for 4 years. His logic was if he changed how he carried his books, people would notice, and he would stand out. I also did things like this when I was at school, keeping my clothes and hair in the same style so I wouldn't attract attention to myself.
- In his final year, Aaron got the courage to carry his books at his side, the same way as the other students.

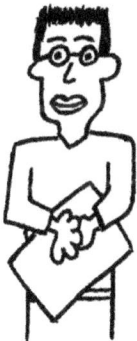

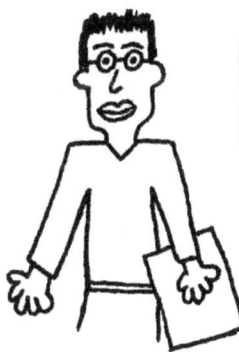

Time Wasters

- Aaron had a job in the library at his university.
- We went to pick him up after work.
- We arrived early so we could see him working. We found him and went over to say 'Hi.'
- He walked straight past us, only his eyes moving, not saying a word.
- Later we said to him, 'You can stop and say Hi.'
- His answer was, 'They don't pay me to socialise.'
- If you want a job done, give it to an Aspie.

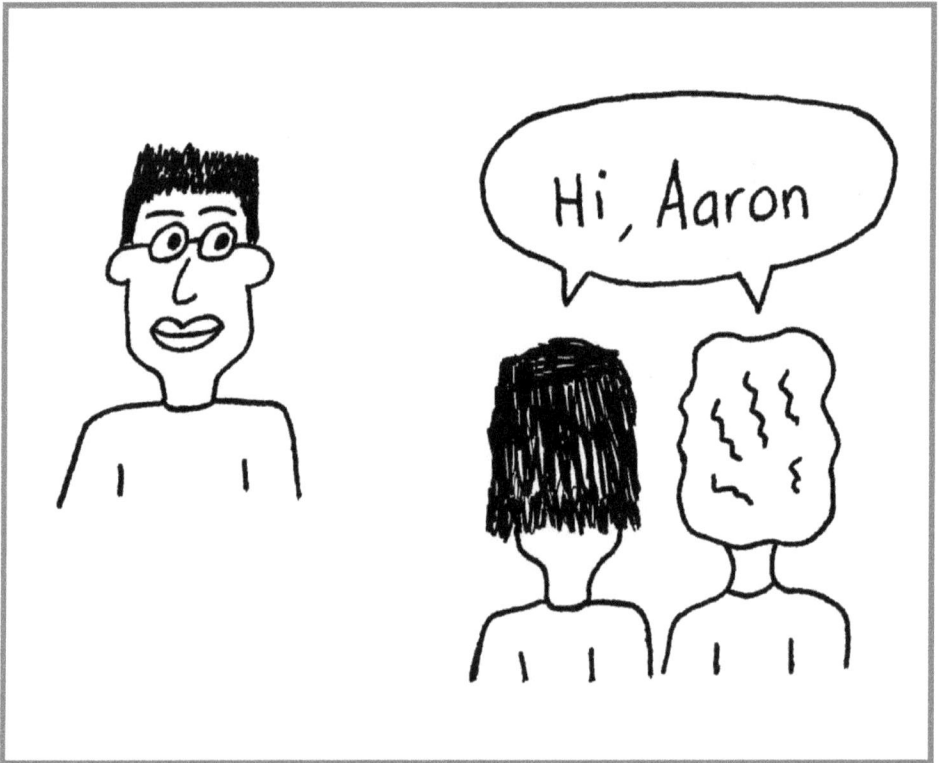

Fight

- When Aaron was growing up, he didn't like to fight back with other kids or have his turn.

- I tried to teach him but never had much luck.

- During his late teens and early twenties, he matured and became more confident, but still didn't have his say.

- As I learned more about Asperger's, I realised I hadn't taught Aaron with clear instructions, I was too vague when he was younger.

- When he was in his mid-twenties, I decided to try an experiment with him.

- Step One - ask Aaron his opinion about himself and then simply agree with him and tell him his opinion was great, even if I didn't believe it. The plan was to build him up to feel that his say was valuable and there would be no repercussions for expressing himself.

- Step Two (many months later) - continue Step One but now occasionally having my say, so that he knows not all his opinions are agreed with.

- Step Three (many months more) - continue Step Two but now I just behave normally, so that we can have a conversation with no one having any issues with other opinions.

- I only moved through the steps when I saw that Aaron was strong enough.

- I just wanted to help Aaron; my way was unique, but my heart was totally involved.

Step One - yeah, yes
Step Two - hmmm, interesting
Step Three - you think What!!!!

Dreams Come True

- At school there are subjects like maths, English and science. To Aspergians, socialising is another subject. We must study it, work at it, and even have 'exams' - trying things out in daily life and feeling like people are judging us, so that even everyday activities feel like a test.

- Aaron has excelled since he left high school. He has two university degrees. He is a volunteer member of a State Emergency Services (SES) unit where he is the administration officer. He also volunteers and acts on the committee for a street market, and volunteers to feed homeless people. He has two groups of friends and is always out socialising. He has a job as a public bus driver, his childhood dream.

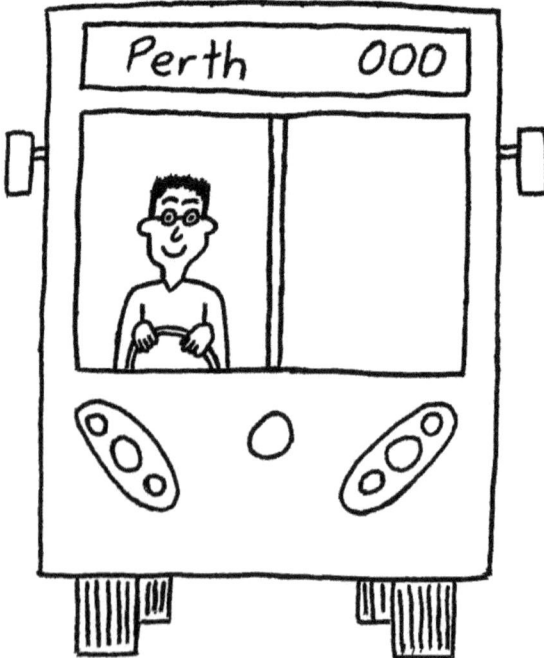

We Are Family

- Oliver was married before and has two adult children; his daughter has three kids. Technically they are my step-grandchildren but that sounds cold and distant - they just know me as Nan, and I love them as my own grandchildren.

- Oliver, Aaron, and I all live together and we have a great relationship. We've always had dogs, who are also a big part of our family.

- Aaron and I talk Aspie and constantly bounce Aspergian knowledge around. Oliver is our link to the social world.

- We all love learning and are very interested in any information one of us can share.

- Our conversations are usually very deep as we work out how the world works in an Aspie way and a neurotypical way.

- We are all do-ers and love trying new things.

- Our household always has humour, and we love having fun.

- We all love each other unconditionally and support each other.

- I am very grateful that I have two people who I can one hundred percent believe in and that Oliver and Aaron can say the same.

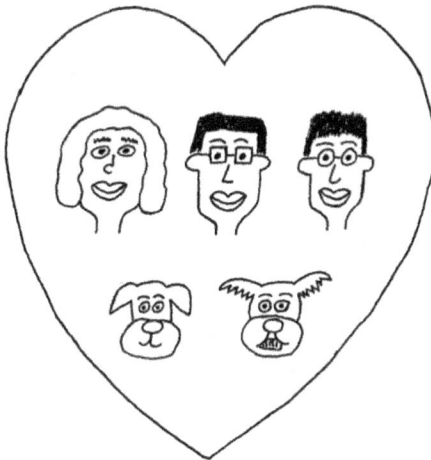

'AND THEN THE STARING BEGINS'

5

WHAT IT'S LIKE BEING ME

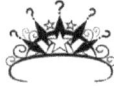

- Monkey Walk
- My Voice
- Brain vs. Mouth
- Clumsy
- Bully
- Stolen Credit
- Day to Day
- Percentages
- Spooky
- Deer in the Headlights
- Time Out

Monkey Walk

- Some interesting things I have learned about Aspergian people:
- The muscle between our thumbs and first finger is not as strong. We therefore have trouble using scissors (noticeable in kindergarten) and our hands get tired after writing for short periods.
- Aspergians tend to hold brushes and toothbrushes like a club.
- Also, Aspies don't use their arms a lot when walking and tend to rock sideways.
- At work there was a guy who liked to imitate me when he saw me walking. He would do a 'Monkey Walk', rocking sideways. He was the only male in our office. I just thought he was stupid and kept away from him.

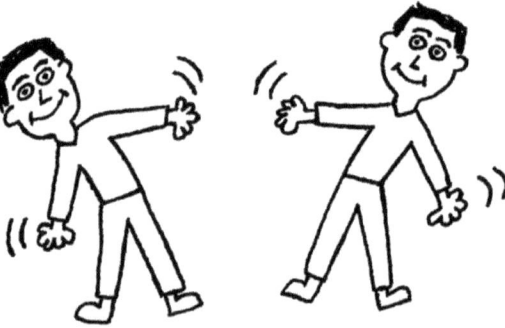

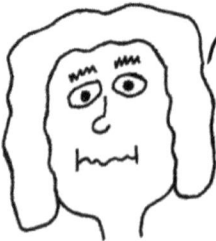

Thinking Back...
Nowadays this would be considered bullying.

My Voice

- My voice seems to do what it wants at times.
- Sometimes I talk in a monotone voice.
- Sometimes my voice goes loud and fast and when I notice, it gets worse, louder, faster and manic.
- My voice is not in my control.

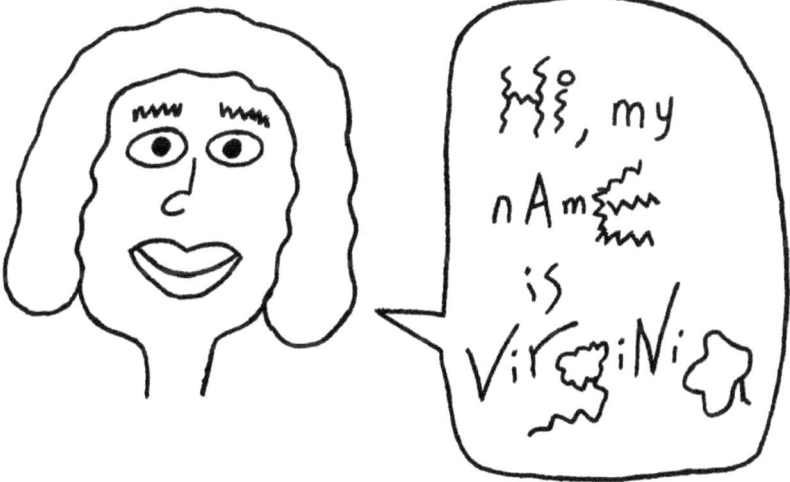

Brain vs. Mouth

- I find my brain and mouth connection is blocked.
- My brain thinks so many thoughts, but I can't get words out of my mouth. My brain goes so fast, my mouth cannot keep up.
- To get my thoughts into words, I need time to process.
- To me I sound stupid as I stumble and um and ah with no actual words coming out.
- My brain has a continuous dialogue going. I am working out all sorts of things all the time, there is never a gap, even when I am meant to be sleeping. It is not stressful to me. I love thinking.
- I can see big words in my head, but I can't get them out. When I try, I find I have invented a new word.
- When people ask me multiple questions, I need to answer the questions in order of asking. My brain cannot keep up and my mouth is silent.

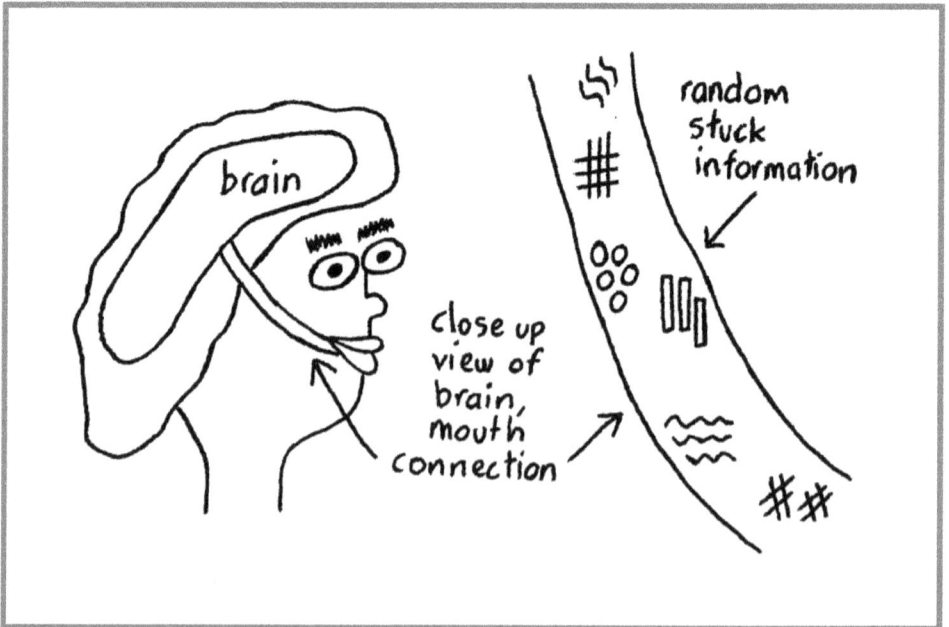

Clumsy

- I am quite a clumsy person.
- I trip over my own feet and walk into walls.
- During aerobics classes, my hands or feet would be in the wrong direction to the other people.
- My speciality is knocking over glasses at tables. I seem to prefer full glasses to empty. People are often grabbing serviettes to help mop up.
- Stepping stones across waterways are tricky. I usually fall in.

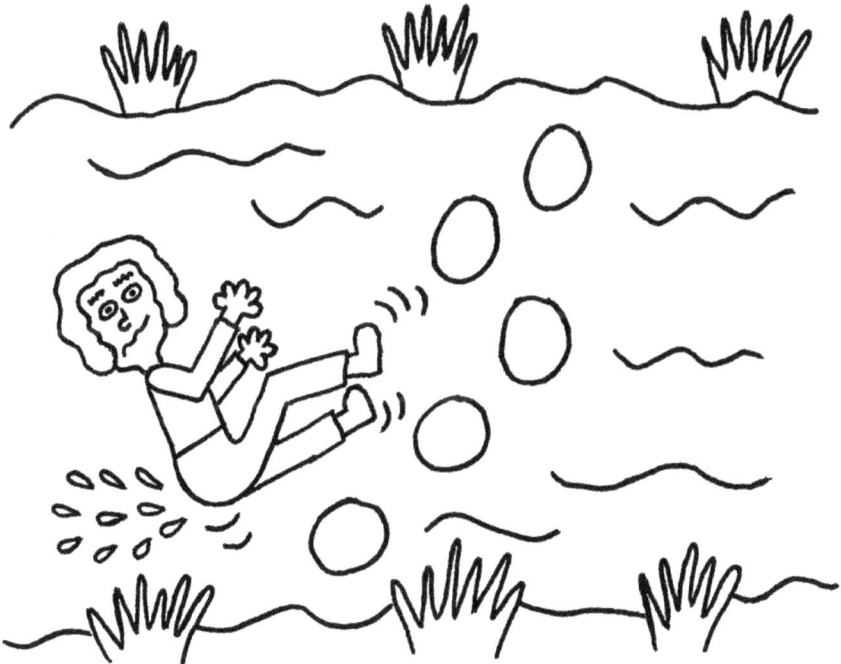

Bully

- Bullies cannot compete with me. I am an expert at being a bully to myself. I rip strips off myself about 'mistakes' I make.
- For example, after socialising, I go through the situation and berate myself that the information I said was not 100% accurate. I want to go back and tell them the correct information.
- I will even beat myself up over things I said or did 20, 30, 40 years ago. Time is no barrier for me.
- I still think people are angry with me from 20 years ago.
- I find that when people try to bully me, it doesn't matter, it is just words. It can only affect me if I attach an emotion to the words.

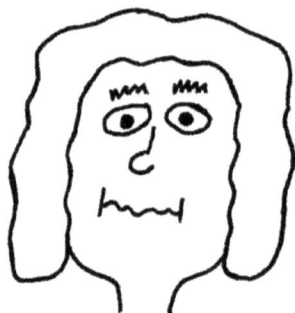

Oh, no, I said there were 16 ducks, there were only 14 ducks

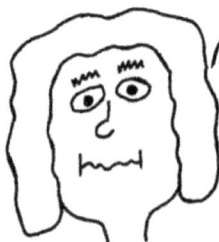

Thinking Back...
I need to look at the positives, not just the negatives. People don't remember day to day, they just don't retain information the way I do.

Stolen Credit

- If someone does something, even something small like come up with an idea and then I get the credit, 'Oh, great idea, Virg,' I will correct them. It is not my credit. I don't want the attention and I feel bad taking the credit.

- If I find someone takes 'stolen credit' and they don't correct it, that is really bad. I know Aspergian people, who when noticing this will be upset and say to me, 'But he didn't do that.'

- Many things Aspies can't be bothered with, like social, but 'stolen credit' – no way.

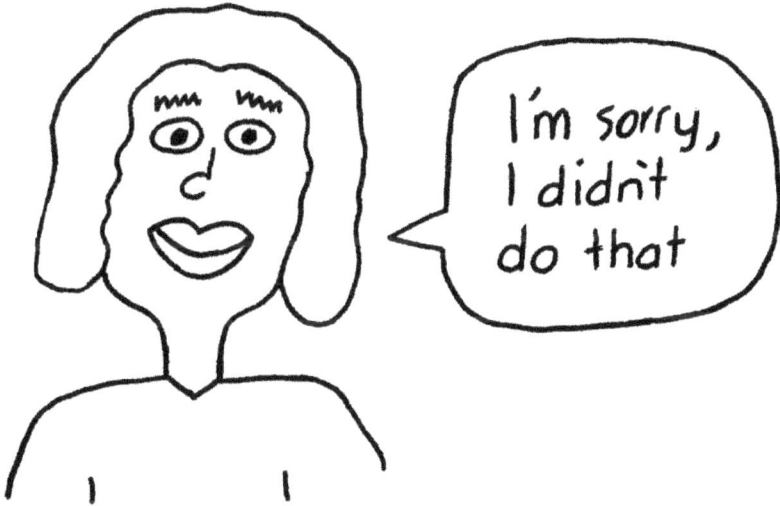

Day to Day

- I can do massive tasks.
- When planning our around-Australia trip, I sat and read for over a year.
- I just divide the task into categories and then complete each category.
- When it comes to day-to-day tasks, however, I have trouble.
- I have things I want to complete, such as floss my teeth, take vitamins, walk the dogs, gym workout, office tasks etc.
- I draw up charts with colours, stickers, rewards points.
- I find if I don't start the day right and miss one task then my whole day is ruined, very black and white thinking.
- I think the main problem is that these tasks are personal, my heart and feelings are involved. They are not detached like the massive tasks I do.
- I also like to have plans for daily jobs e.g., cleaning. I divide the tasks into a list, such as 'Dining room – clear clutter, dust, sweep, mop'. I mark off the tasks as I go along.
- Even if I go to the shops, I plan the journey in my head - which shops I'm going to and what I am buying.

Tuesday 7 May
· floss ✓
· vitamins ✓
· pay bills ✓
· treadmill x
· wash dogs ✓
· wash clothes x

Wednesday 8 May
· floss
· vitamins
· accounts
· walk dogs
· food shop

Percentages

- Many things Oliver does confuse me. My black and white thinking kicks in.

- In the days before mobile phones, Oliver would say he was just going down to the shops to buy bread. The shops are less than a kilometre from our house. He would return three hours later, and I would be frantic. 'Where have you been?' I would ask. He would say, 'Oh, I also went to the hardware shop and the chemist.' He hadn't told me that he was going to do those things.

- Sometimes he says he will do something for me, then he gets side-tracked. I will be waiting and waiting, getting more and more annoyed, thinking he is ignoring me on purpose, paying me back for something I did to him before.

- Another example is when he leaves his shoes in the doorway of our bedroom, so that I have to step over them. I believe he has done it on purpose, again as payback, trying to make me trip over. When he says he didn't do it on purpose, I think he is lying.

- When I explain that I think he is being 100% evil to me on purpose, he knows it is my black/white thinking. He puts things into a percentage: he can't possibly be 100% evil, look at all the nice things he does for me.

- I agree, he is just 51% evil.

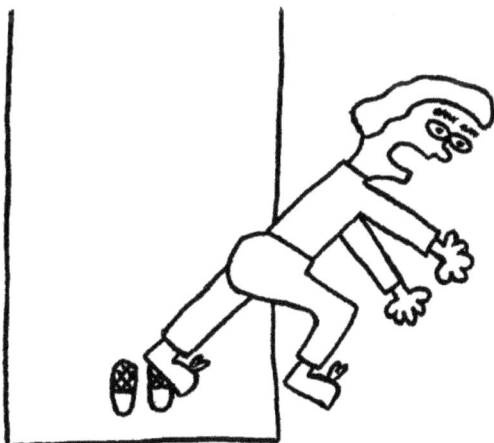

Spooky

- I seem to be able to see and feel spooky things.

- Once when walking past a headstone in a cemetery, I suddenly felt an evil energy and when I kept walking it disappeared. It was coming from just that one headstone.

- When walking around a cathedral, there was one spot where I felt all tingly and heavy. I walked around the whole cathedral once more, returned to the same spot and felt it again, just that one spot. I researched the cathedral's floor plan and found that the spot was near a crypt where priests' bodies were laid.

- I have found on numerous occasions when I'm requesting something on the phone and the answer is no, I can send energy so the answer will change to yes. For example, Oliver and I phoned a caravan park for a site. The receptionist answered 'Oh, I'm sorry, we are fully booked.' I sent her an energy wave. 'Oh, hold on, I've just been told that a mistake was made and there's one site. That wasn't there this morning.'

- When we were in Italy, there was a historic walkway built on top of a church. The railings were very low, and I felt an immense desire to throw myself off the building. I stayed low and knew it wasn't me, it was an evil energy. Later I found out that many people in historic times had met their deaths there.

- When at crowded places, I will surround myself with positive energy so that people will feel calm around me. It works.

- When Oliver's mum was in hospital and the family were advised she would pass on, all the family members gathered around her bed. I was at the door (the room was very crowded) and when she died, I had a feeling to look up. I saw her spirit there, leaning over a small wall, looking down with a confused face. I think she was wondering what was going on. I wasn't scared, just intrigued.

- Oliver's dad died at home. I felt like going into his bedroom. I could feel his spirit there. I asked Oliver to come into the room, without telling him why. In the room, Oliver's face and neck suddenly burst into goose bumps, looking like plucked chicken skin. Oliver's body reacted but his brain did not – now that is spooky.

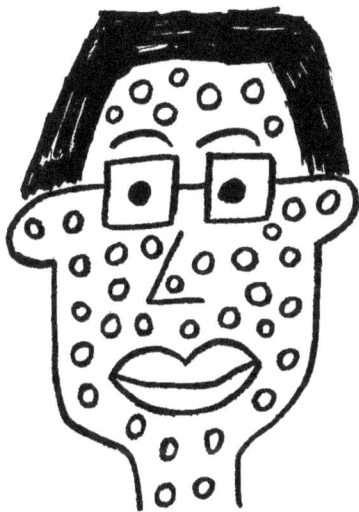
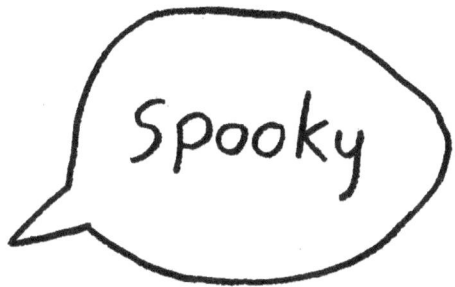

Deer in the Headlights

- I often stand and look at people like a 'deer in the headlights', just staring at the person, not knowing what to say or do.

- When someone is yelling at me, I just stare and watch. I'm not listening to their words, just watching them. The more I stare, the angrier they get.

- Other times when I am asked a question but don't know if it is a question, I will just stare until I know I am expected to answer.

- When meeting people that I barely know in the shops, they ask me, 'How have you been?' I answer, 'Good' and then the staring begins. They ask, 'What have you been up to?', more staring. My brain is going full speed, asking myself questions such as 'What do they really want to know?', 'What are their intentions?', 'Are they asking me a question?', 'Are they manipulating me for their own benefit?'

- I eventually answer with a brief response, but I am very aware that I look startled. I probably look like I am trying to hide something from them.

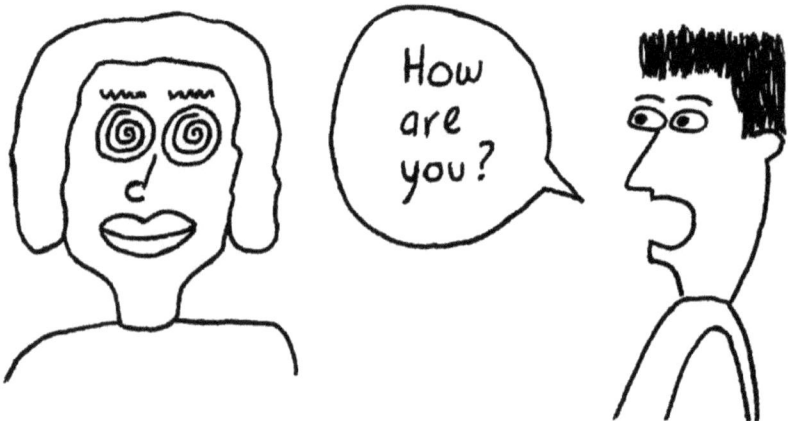

Time Out

- For me, socialising is work.
- I am always thinking about what to say, what not to say, how I stand or how I sit. It gets tiring.
- I need time out to stay home in my predictable environment.
- Sometimes I just like to read books all day.
- Oliver is very much aware of this and knows too much social is stressful for both Aaron and me.
- I love being in my house with Oliver, Aaron, and the dogs, we all get along together so well.
- It doesn't matter what we say or do, we all support each other unconditionally.

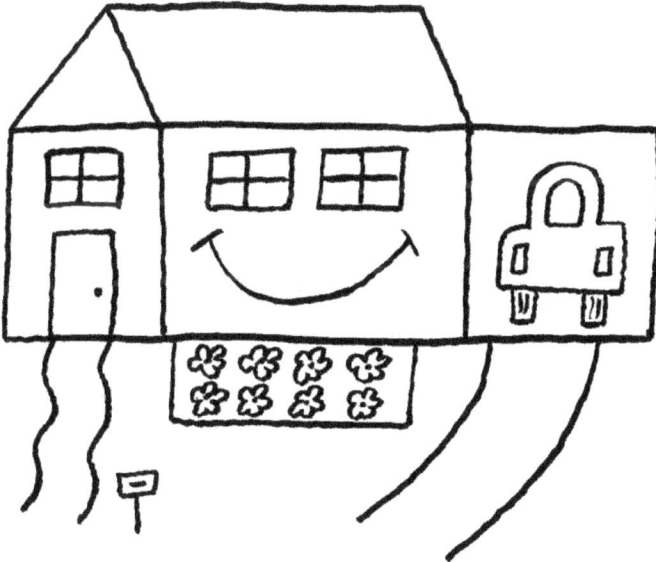

'IT FEELS AS IF MY SKIN IS MOVING'

6

SENSORY AND FEELINGS

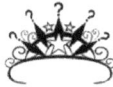

- Senses
- Empathy
- Super Aware
- Audio
- Change
- Emotions
- Obsessive Compulsive Disorder
- Touching and Sex
- Town Hall
- Meltdown

Senses

- My senses are all heightened. I am very aware of my surroundings.
- Concerts and basketball games are too loud for me. I wear earplugs.
- Some languages are pleasant to listen to and some languages get me so agitated that I need to block my ears.
- I don't like jazz or electric guitars, wrong frequencies.
- Strong perfume odours hurt my throat and choke me.
- I hear and smell things before other people do and point it out to them.
- I love details that are still, and I can enjoy the patterns, but moving details such as action movies or cities are very stressful. I feel like I am being punched in the face.
- Touch is a big issue. I don't like strangers to touch me, especially massages. My neck and shoulders tense up and it feels as if my skin is moving. I shake and twitch just thinking about it. The feel of beach sand is bad. Just thinking about it makes my legs all tingly.
- If I am stressed, Oliver can't touch me, my skin feels super sensitive. When I am not stressed, I like to cuddle and touch people I like. If I don't like someone, I find their touch difficult and I need to shake and wipe their touch off me afterwards.
- My neck is totally off limits (the same with Aaron and my dad).
- When I have a shower, my face must be dry. I always have a towel handy.
- Note: Aaron was as tall as the swimming instructor before he passed Level One because he didn't want water on his face.

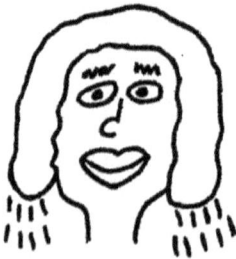

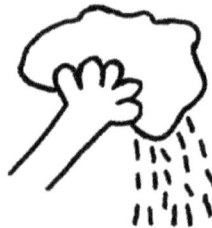

nice
dry
face

Empathy

- I believe there are two types of empathy.
- The first is when you 'step into the other person's shoes', meaning you feel what they feel.
- The second is when someone hurts themselves, your heart goes out to them. You want to help them.
- I find it easy to 'step into someone else's shoes'.
- When people or animals are hurt, I have a problem. I feel too much, all the suffering, the screaming, the injustice. It is too much and I shut down. I cannot hold that much inside me.
- If I am not overwhelmed by my feelings when something is happening, I can help others. If I am depleted emotionally, I have no more to give, I can't help.
- I can't give false sympathy or pretend to care.
- I don't like helping people who I know are being nasty.
- If I see other people genuinely helping others, I get emotional and cry. I feel the love.

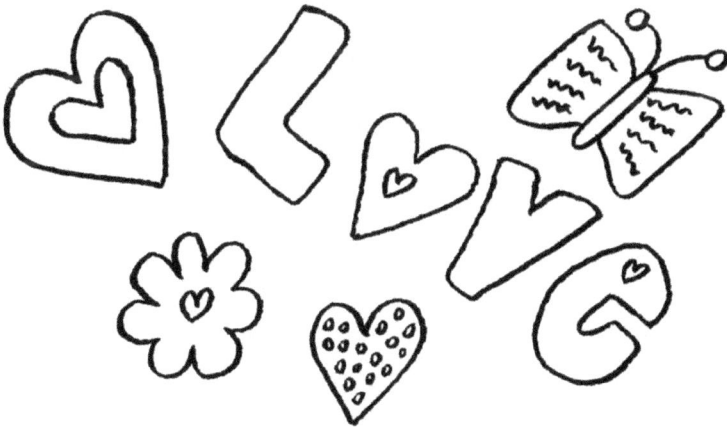

Super Aware

- I find when I am in public that my awareness level is super high.
- I concentrate on my breathing, how I walk, the feeling of my clothes against my body.
- When I eat, I notice that I concentrate on my chewing.
- Once, at a formal birthday party where everyone was sitting at tables, I saw someone I know who has Asperger's.
- He was walking very stiffly, as if he had an ironing board up his shirt. His arms were straight down, not moving, and his eyes were darting about while his head was perfectly still. He was so aware of himself, so stressed out.

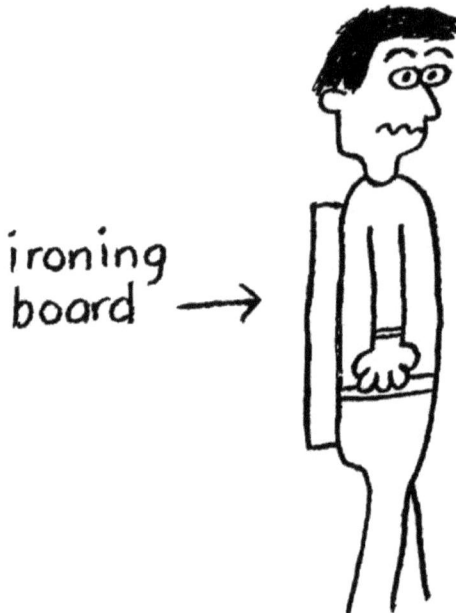

ironing board →

Audio

- I get a lot of information - and irritation - from audio.

- I love to repeat interesting sounds or words out loud. I love the patterns the sounds and words make.

- I can't have two audio sources going on at once, e.g., TV and radio. It is very stressful, my heartbeat increases.

- When watching TV, I get way more information from the audio. I am usually reading or doing puzzles because I don't need to see all the visuals.

- I hear all the background noises wherever I am. For example, in a restaurant I hear the cutlery and talking from other tables, the kitchen sounds, chairs, and plates scraping. It is only stressful if I need to concentrate on one sound amid all the noise.

- If I don't get an audio response or people are not facing me, I don't know what to do e.g., I was once telling a story to a group of people around a picnic table. At first some people were looking at me, then they all were looking away making their lunch. I did not know what to do, e.g., do I continue the story, it will be weird if I suddenly stop. I kept going and people laughed at the right times, so OK.

- When people say things to me, I need to repeat what they said out loud (I try to keep the volume down). It is like I need to hear the words from my own mouth to understand them.

- I find I must keep repeating the same question to people if I don't get an audible answer. I don't know if the person has heard me. I can't read the body language.

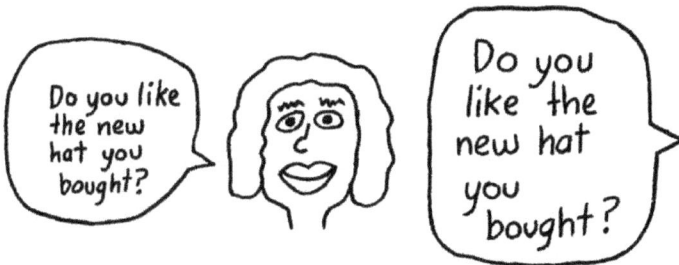

Do you like the new hat you bought?

Do you like the new hat you bought?

Change

- I don't like change.

- If I am doing an activity and I must stop because someone else's activity is taking place, it really agitates me. I want to complete my task, and to complete tasks in order.

- When people plan something, I will stick to the plan only to find that they are not, they changed their minds. That really annoys me; there is no structure, it's just aimless.

- If something is often done a certain way, I know the outcome. I don't like a new way, not knowing what the outcome will be.

- I like things in my house to stay in the same place so I can just go there and grab what I want and not have to search for it.

- If part of an activity must be rearranged, it really agitates me. I have that part of the activity already organised in my head.

- When things change, I find I don't breathe, I need to move around, my heartbeat goes fast, and I get bossy.

- One time we got a new (second-hand) fridge. I worried for a few days; I couldn't find things. I was explaining my uneasiness to Oliver and Aaron. Then Aaron looked at my shoes (brand new) and said, 'I like your new shoes.' Well, that shook me back to reality.

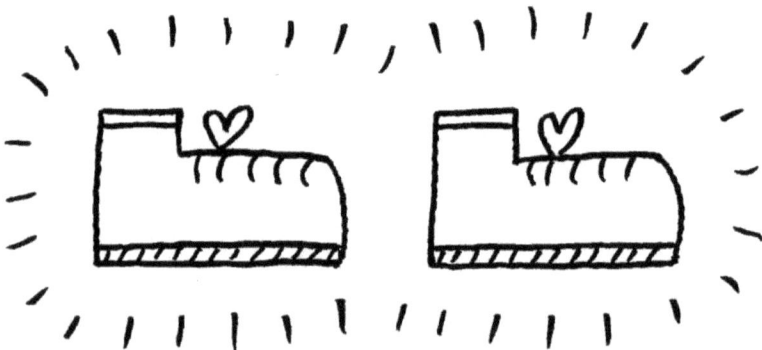

Emotions

- I like to use my emotions fully, e.g., if I am happy, I show happy.
- People often watch me, some amused, some shocked and some get excited with me.
- My emotions are already on a high and I don't have much room to move. I hit extreme quite fast, then when I react, it is full-on.
- I find I am always fidgeting, emotions ready.
- With my emotions there are usually body reactions such as shaking and crying.
- I remember a family visit to the zoo. I was already on alert. At the zoo there were crowds, strong smells, lots of different noises at different levels. I kept myself under control, but I was very aware, and my emotions were stressed out.

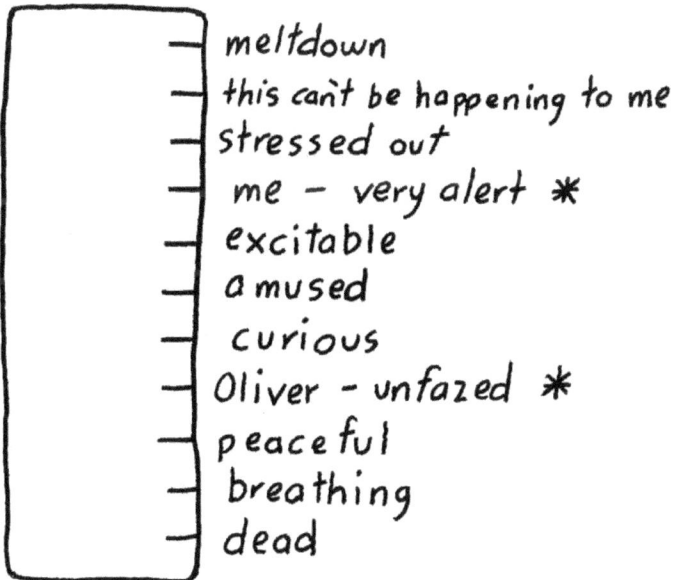

meltdown
this can't be happening to me
stressed out
me – very alert *
excitable
amused
curious
Oliver – unfazed *
peaceful
breathing
dead

Obsessive Compulsive Disorder

- I believe my OCD started when Aaron was a small child.

- OCD means I must do restrictive, repetitive actions. I fear that something bad will happen if I don't.

- With laundry, I must hang the clothes in a certain direction and right way up. Also, the same colour peg can't be next to each other.

- During the day, there are many times I have trouble picking out an item; it can be anything. I have many pairs of socks, sometimes it is impossible to choose, and they all begin to look evil, so I just get Oliver to pick a pair. It can be a pair I picked out earlier, but that is OK because I trust Oliver's choice - he knows which pair is not evil.

- Another issue is if I have a bowl or plate of food. I don't want people to touch my food, they have germs and I put that food in my mouth. If it does happen, I separate the touched food.

- Feelings of stress can send me into OCD thinking, especially on holidays. Should I choose the left or right walking path? How should I pack the suitcase? Which grapes on my plate are evil? When I know this is happening, I tell myself off. I don't have magical powers that can cause bad things to happen just because I walked to the left of a pillar instead of on the right.

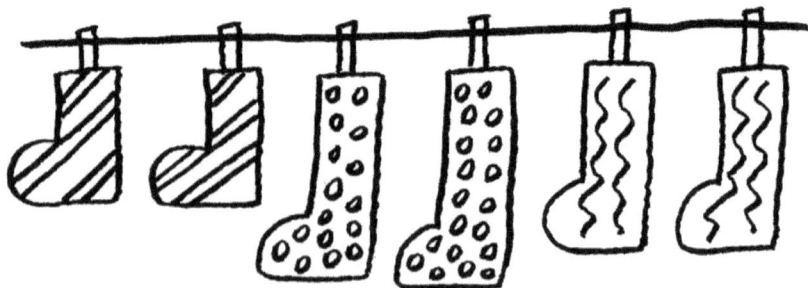

Touching and Sex

- Physical affection was very important for Oliver when he was growing up. His parents and uncles and aunties were always touching him with love.

- My childhood was so different. I rarely experienced safe, affectionate physical contact.

- 'First Friend' showed me about affectionate touching and I liked it.

- Oliver and I were always holding hands, sitting close next to each other and hugging. Friends would get annoyed with us, saying 'You two are always on top of each other, can't you leave each other alone.'

- There is no shyness with my body with Oliver because my logic says that once Oliver has seen everything then there is nothing to hide anymore.

- When it comes to sex, we have no special routines, it is just like other people – Part A goes into Slot B, repeat, repeat, repeat, etc.

- With Oliver I have learned that physical affection can be calming and safe.

- When I go to doctors or psychologists, Oliver is always with me because I have no secrets with him, I am very comfortable with him and I know that he loves to learn any new information, just like me.

- Touching and affection are so normal for Aaron. Aunties were especially enthusiastic with cuddles. Aaron would just stand there, smiling and receiving. We taught him that giving and receiving affection is normal and safe in our family.

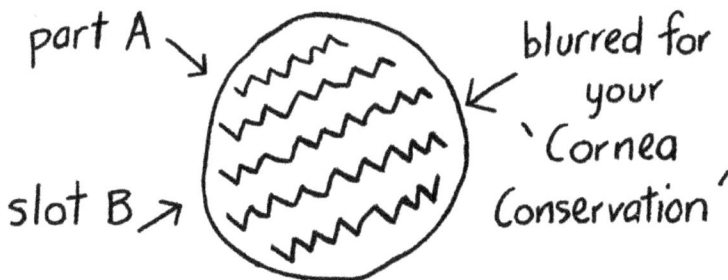

part A
slot B
blurred for your 'Cornea Conservation'

Town Hall

- Age: 50
- Oliver and I went to a birthday party at the Town Hall in the city.
- The Town Hall was packed with guests sitting around round tables.
- There were all kinds of different acts on the stage for our entertainment.
- When dinner was served, the acts stopped, and background music was turned on.
- I felt my body relax, all the tension came out of my shoulders and neck, and I was breathing normally again. I had been holding my breath and not breathing properly during the two hours of the entertainment acts. During the acts, I was not aware that I was doing this.
- The problem was the massive echo in the room from the microphones. The audio was so stressful, not knowing where the sounds were coming from, bouncing around the room.

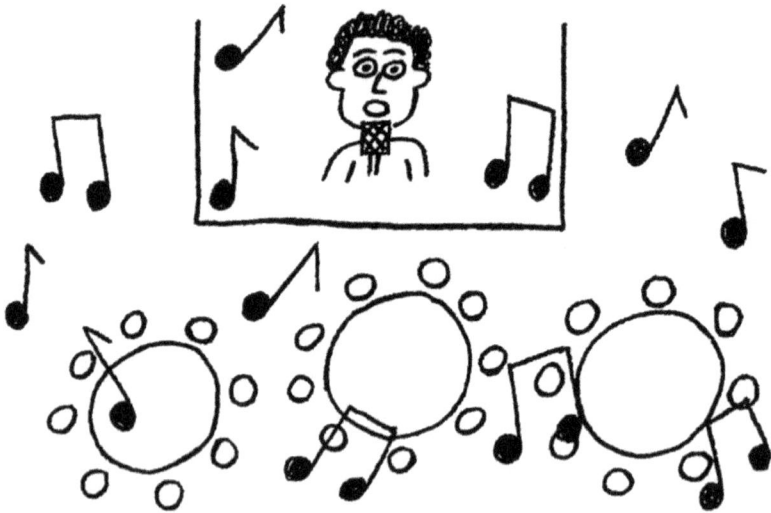

Meltdown

- Age: late 50s
- When I have too many emotions and sensory issues, I can have a meltdown. I have had many meltdowns, but never really analysed the feelings until the following event occurred:
- I was shopping with Oliver during an overseas holiday when we received an emotional email from a friend back in Perth who wasn't coping.
- This really threw me. We sent a supportive message back, but I was so concerned.
- After shopping, we went to a food hall. There was so much noise, different languages, people too close to me and horrible smells.
- Back at the hotel, I was so emotional, crying on and off.
- That night we had a huge social event (outdoor concert) to attend. I was so overwhelmed; where was I going to stand, what about the noise, the smells, the people bumping into me.
- I couldn't go, I was just too emotional, jumpy and very agitated.
- The next day, I was super aware of my surroundings, the footpath, the other people, the traffic. I was trying to act like I usually did but I noticed I was over-acting; super aware, trying to control every aspect of myself, the way I walked and talked, my body position, my breathing, my eyes, the friction of my clothes. I knew I looked weird.
- The following day I realized I had experienced a meltdown.
- I needed a time-out day.

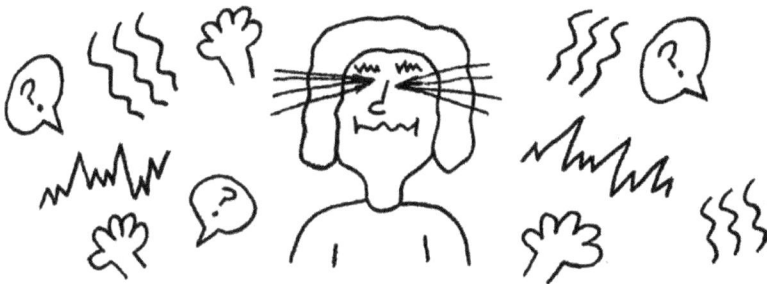

'I'M ASPERGIAN / MENOPAUSAL NOT NUTS'

7

DIAGNOSIS

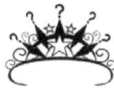

- Insane
- Menopause
- Diagnosis

Insane

- Age: mid 40s
- The world was so confusing to me.
- I started to worry about my sanity, I just couldn't understand people. I didn't know about Asperger's.
- It seemed I was always annoying people, and they would be angry with me.
- People were constantly lying, saying things like 'I'll come over', 'I'd love to borrow that', 'I'll phone you'. So, I would get ready, and then they wouldn't turn up.
- People didn't obey any rules.
- I just seemed to do things in a different way to others.
- People didn't want me to tell them the truth.
- I would open my heart to others just so they could stab it.
- Why would someone be nice to me and then ignore me next time?
- I was anxious, confused, and worried.
- I was finally diagnosed in 2014 at the age of 49.
- I wasn't insane, I was Aspergian.

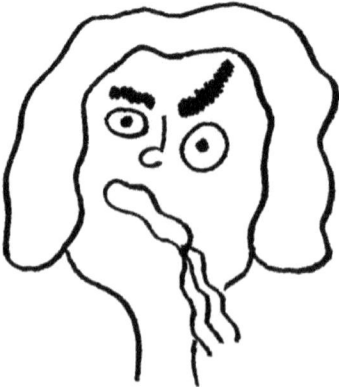

me, insane

Menopause

- Age: mid 50s
- Menopause has been hard.
- My Aspergian qualities have all doubled.
- I feel like I have PMT (pre-menstrual tension) every day. I am angry and emotional, crying one minute and happy the next.
- My sleeping, which has never been great, is now about two hours a night.
- Childhood fears have come back. I never felt safe as a child - there was no security in my life. Menopause messes with my thoughts - I find myself checking under beds and behind doors for people who want to harm me.
- The sweats make it look like I have a permanent shower above my head.
- My mind has not been right. All the mood swings and brain fogs.
- The worst thing is finding a doctor who has enough knowledge to help. As soon as I mention that my mind is not right, the doctor wants me to see a psychiatrist. I am Aspergian/menopausal, not nuts.

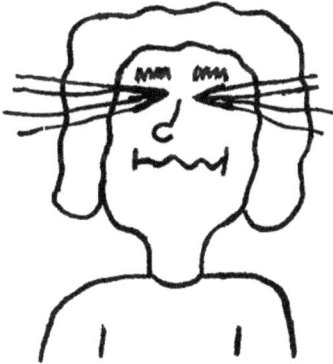

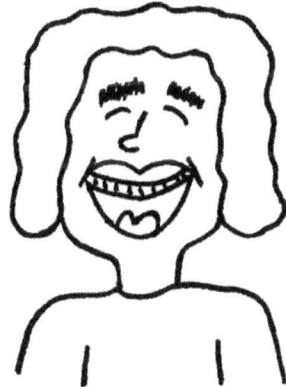

one minute later

Diagnosis

- Age: 49
- Like many Aspergian women, I was diagnosed after my child was identified as having Autism Spectrum Disorder. This is how many women get diagnosed - their child is assessed as having ASD, the parents start researching and discover the similarities. Many girls and women are not diagnosed because they are very good at copying others, masking their ASD symptoms.
- In supporting Aaron, Oliver and I came into contact with many professionals and organisations involved with ASD. That is how I met Winnie. I made an appointment with her and at the age of forty-nine I was diagnosed with Asperger's.
- Having the diagnosis gave me the answers about why I do things my way. I could now research and learn. It is like when you have an illness and suffer. When you know what you have you can get correct medication and help yourself. Before that, you feel helpless.
- I love having Asperger's, that I think differently and am not hindered by 'social' - I am not a sheep, following by peer pressure.
- When I was labelled as someone with a traumatic childhood, it meant I was a victim and would have to work through issues to heal but having Asperger's means I am unique and have power. I don't have to fix anything, I can just learn how to adapt to the social world.
- If I had been labelled as insane, it would also have meant that I had no power. I was truly worried that I was going to end up in a mental hospital. Asperger's = power. I was just thinking differently to others, and I liked that. I could embrace my differences, which are my true core. I am independent.
- Also, when I understood about hyperthymesia, I discovered that it is rare to have excessive memory and realised that maybe I shouldn't hassle other people for not remembering things.
- For me, Asperger's and hyperthymesia means I have superpowers. I should probably wear my undies on the outside.

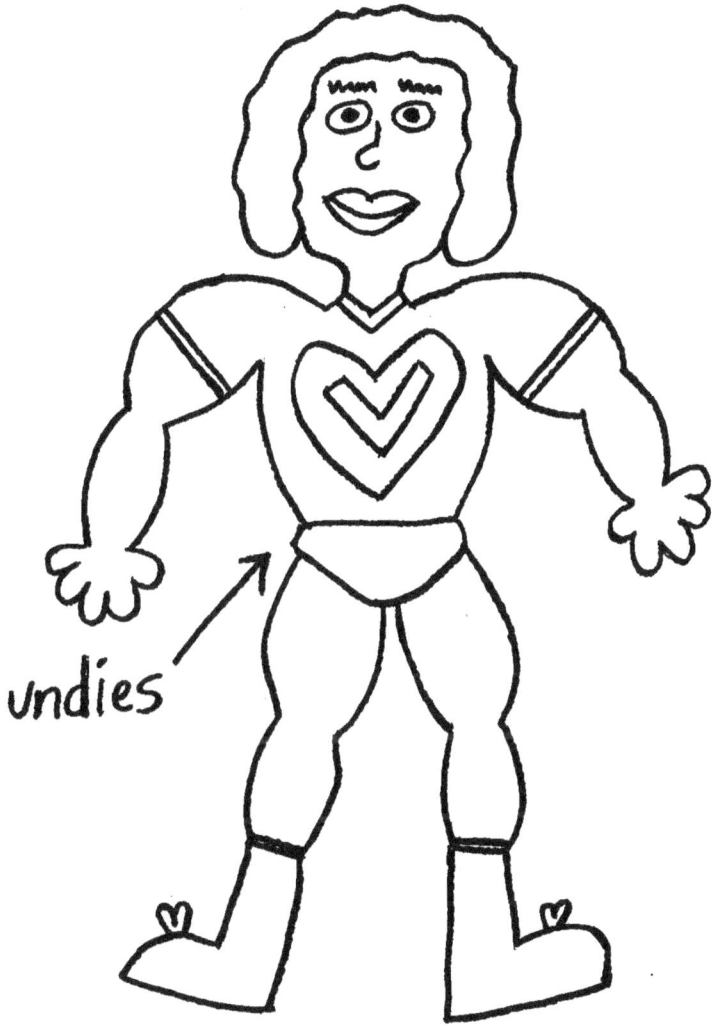

undies

'I WOULD OPEN MY HEART FULLY'

8

READING PEOPLE

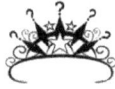

- Facing Off
- One View
- Porn Star
- Your Local Weather Reporter
- New Best Friend
- Which Page?

Facing Off

- When looking at people's faces, I don't like very much eye contact. I find it overly personal, as though people can see into my soul. I also feel that it's too close, too sexual for me.
- I feel people can see my secrets, but after this book that problem will be solved!
- During a conversation, I get all my information from the person's mouth, like a lip reader. The rest of the face tells me nothing.
- I am also very big on 'tone of voice'. I can hear if people are lying, nervous, excited, manipulating, emotional. The tone tells me a lot.

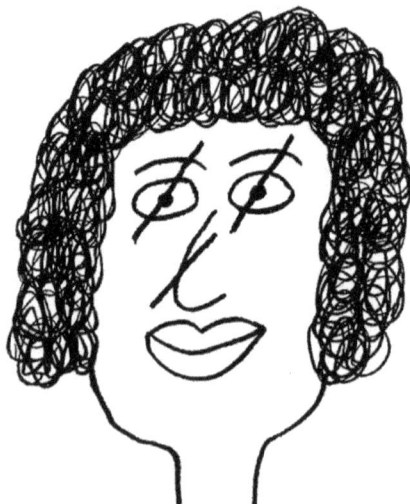

/ = no information

One View

- I showed Oliver a picture of children playing outside and eating watermelon slices.
- I asked him what he saw, and he answered, 'Kids having fun' and that he felt happy.
- He said he saw the picture as a whole.
- What I saw were the details. My eyes locked onto the red watermelon slices, and I counted the black seeds.
- My only emotion was feeling disturbed when I noticed that one of the watermelon slices had only three seeds, not four.
- My eyes then spread over the picture, and I saw a child climbing a tree.
- I saw the picture in individual pieces.
- I realised the same applied when people talked to Oliver and me.
- When Oliver listens to someone, the words join together to give each sentence an overall meaning.
- Unlike Oliver, I latch on to individual details or words; this can totally change my understanding.
- For example: A person says to me, 'I can accommodate you with a car.' I answer, 'But I was going to stay in a hotel.' Person, annoyed: 'I don't care where you stay, I can accommodate you with a car.' Me, becoming upset because I don't want to sleep in a car: 'But I have already paid for the hotel.' Person, angry: 'Is this a joke, do you want the car or not?' Me, very upset, through tears: 'Of course I want the car, I just have to cancel the hotel first.'
- I get so obsessed with the one word, in this example the word 'accommodate', which I take to mean a place to sleep, that I get stuck, and I can't move on.
- Some people who know me work out that I have misunderstood one word, and they calmly direct me to the correct meaning of the whole sentence.

Porn Star

- Age: late 20s
- I found a breast lump (it turned out to be just a cyst).
- I told my doctor and he said, 'I'll need to have a look at that.' He turned around to his desk and when he turned back to me, I was naked from the waist up.
- He had a very surprised face.

Reading Faces:
What I thought the doctor might be thinking...

A. Oh, I forgot to buy eggs.
B. Wow, those are big.
C. Why does she have no clothes on?

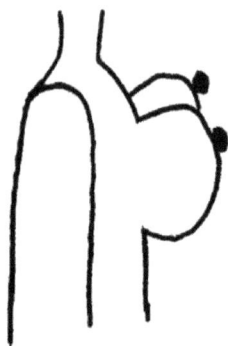

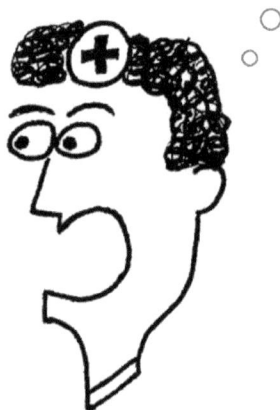

Answer:
At the time, I thought it was B. The answer is probably C.

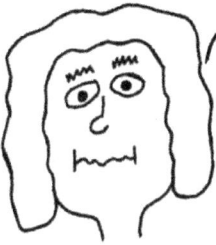

Thinking Back...
The doctor would probably have organised a nurse, got me to put on a gown in private, and have me lie down on the bed.

Your Local Weather Reporter

- Age: 40s
- I was putting my groceries through the checkout.
- The checkout chick asked me, 'What's the weather like outside?' I had a good think, trying to remember and not wanting to get the answer wrong. I said, 'It is sunny.'
- When I got outside, it was raining, so I ran back to her to report the updated weather.
- She pulled a constipated face and I thought, 'Oh no, there go her afternoon plans.'

Reading Faces:
What I thought the checkout chick might be thinking...

A. All my afternoon plans are destroyed.
B. I need to go to the toilet so bad.
C. Why is she talking to me, why is she here?

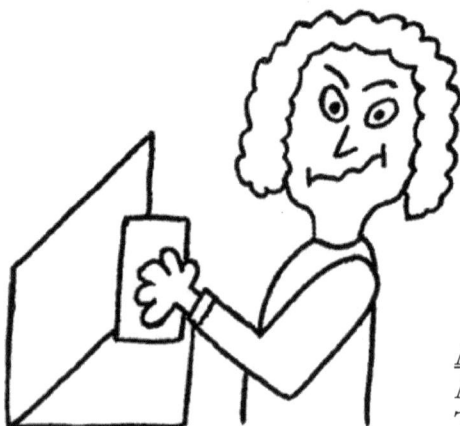

Answer:
At the time, I thought it was A.
The answer is probably C.

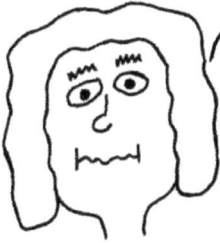

Thinking Back...
Her question about the weather was just friendly small talk, like a longer way of saying Hello.

New Best Friend

- I used to have a naïve response when a total stranger was nice to me: I would open my heart fully to them.

- But the next time I met them they would be cold towards me, and it hurt.

- One time at a caravan park, the office lady was so nice, and we were talking and laughing. I felt so close to her, my heart so open. I wanted to hang out with her afterwards.

- The next day, I went to the office, and I was so excited to see her. She acted like she had never met me. She was neutral and not friendly at all.

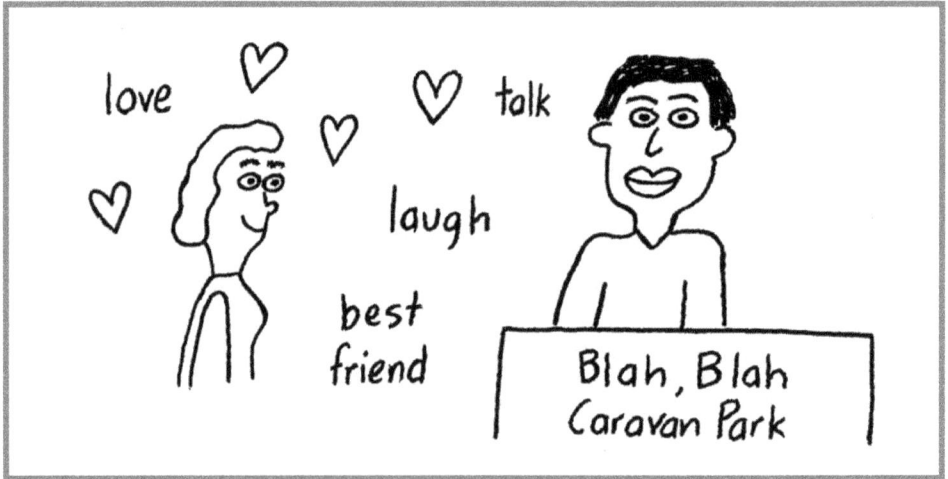

love ♡ ♡ talk
♡ ♡
laugh
best
friend
Blah, Blah
Caravan Park

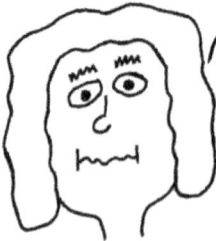

Thinking Back...
I know now that if a stranger is friendly, just enjoy that one time because they are simply being social. I know next time not to expect the same response from them.

Which Page?

- Age: late 50s
- I was walking home and near my house one set of neighbours were outside looking at a water mains.
- The neighbours on the other side of the road came home and the two sets of neighbours started talking to each other from across the road.
- I didn't know what to do as I walked up to the neighbours. My mind was flipping through my 'Social Manual' to find the page that this situation was on.
- I looked in the direction of one of the neighbours, but they were so intensely talking that they did not notice me.
- I just walked on past them and into my house, next door, not saying anything.
- At home, I explained the situation to Oliver and that I was trying to find the right page (in my mind) for the rules. He said, 'It is on page one, just say Hello.'
- I couldn't see this. The situation was not the same as anything I had been in before, the rules are not transferrable to me, I need a new set of rules for a new situation.
- Once again Oliver highlighted how simple social life is for neurotypicals.

Page One

Rule: say `Hello'

This technique can be applied to ALL situations

'**I WENT DRESSED AS A POO**'

9

THAT'S HOW I AM

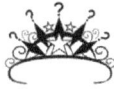

- Points of View
- P Parties
- What's in a Name?
- Ahead of the Pack
- Girls and Guys
- Instinct
- Bloody Tea
- Taboo Shops

Points of View

- Our local pool had a 5-metre outdoor diving platform.
- I was wearing my new white bikini (wet from previous swimming) and was standing at the very top of the platform.
- What a view, I could see for miles. No one was waiting, so I stayed up there a while trying to locate my house.
- When I dived in and swam to my friend, she said, 'Do you know your bikini is see-through?'
- What a view.

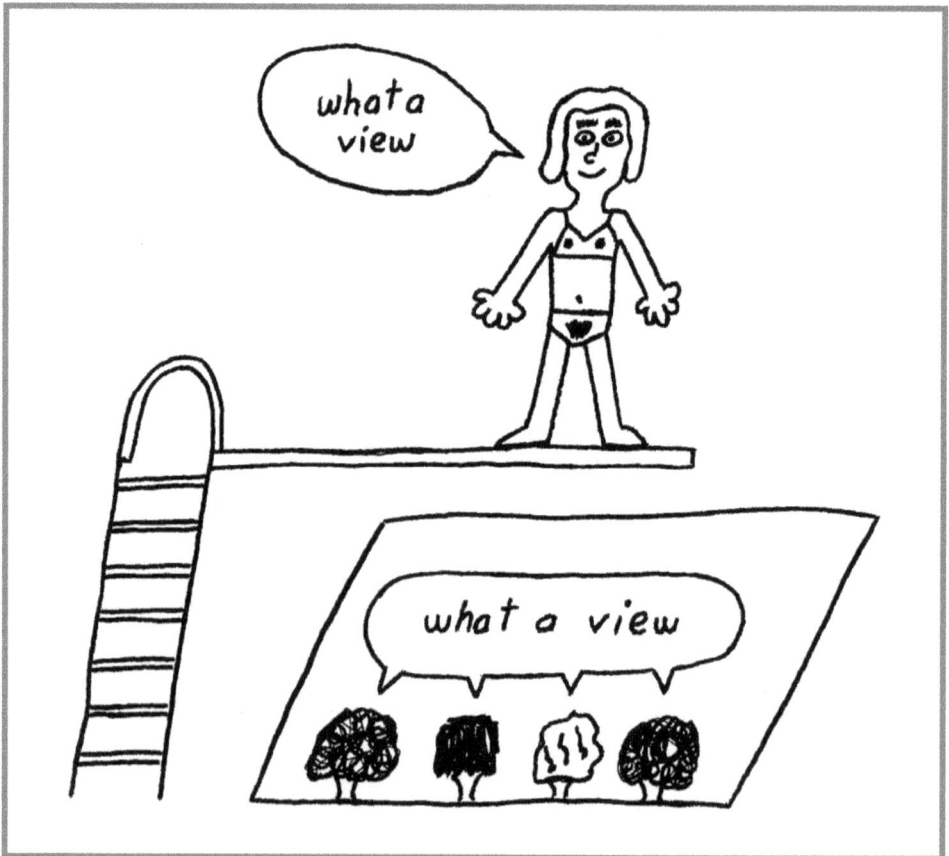

P Parties

- I have been to two 'P' parties where you dress up as something beginning with the letter P.
- My first party, I went dressed as a 'Poo'. I made a long brown costume, from my head to hanging down between my legs. It did look like a poo.
- People were amused by my poo costume and joked that it smelled, which made me laugh.
- The second party, I went as a urine sample ('Pee').
- Oliver helped me make the costume. He surrounded me with a firm plastic sheet and a black cardboard top. On the plastic he drew froth.
- Other people at the party were shocked by my costume.
- Oliver would have dressed in something very conservative that we can't even remember.

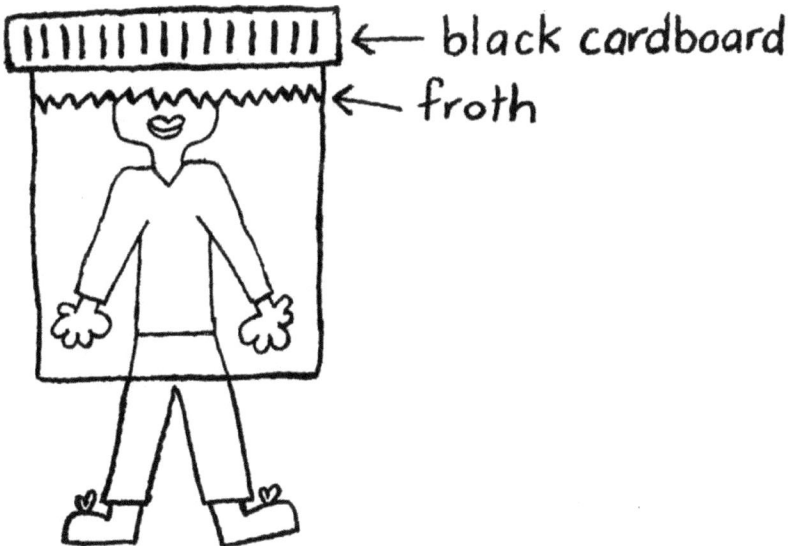

← black cardboard

← froth

What's in a Name?

- I have my hair cut at a 'shearing shed' style hairdressing shop. Many of the hairdressers are backpacking travellers from Europe, and English is not their first language.

- One day, after having my name written down at reception, I waited in the waiting area, which was full of people.

- Next thing, the backpacker/hairdresser looks in the book and yells out, 'Vagina, Vagina.' I knew it was me, but I was not going to stand up in a packed waiting area to 'Vagina'.

- The manager rushed over to her (maybe yelling out 'Vagina, Vagina' is bad for business) and then calls my name, 'Virginia'. I jump up and say to myself, 'Yes, people, that is my name.'

- Another haircut event was in the 1980s when big hair was the fashion.

- After my haircut, the hairdresser teased, frizzed, and tossed my hair into a massive messy mountain. She asked me, 'How do you like it?'

- I answered, 'Well usually it takes the whole night in bed, tossing and turning to get it to look like that.'

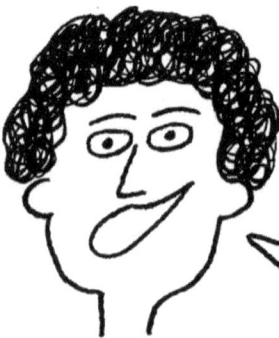

Ahead of the Pack

- Age: early 20s
- A strange thing happened when I went to see the movie *Naked Gun* starring Leslie Nielson.
- I went by myself and sat at the side of the theatre.
- The movie has my type of humour, and I understood the jokes very quickly. I would see the joke and laugh.
- Then there was an echo when the rest of the people in the theatre would start to laugh.
- This happened all through the movie, the delayed second laughter.

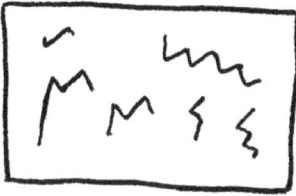

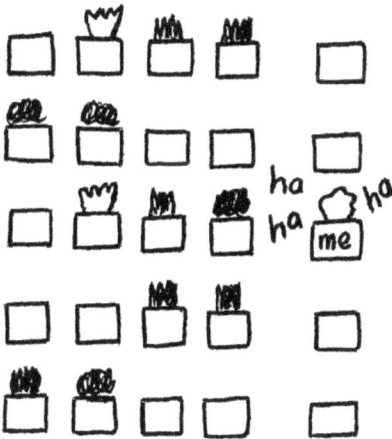

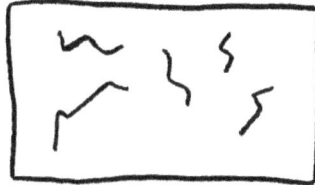

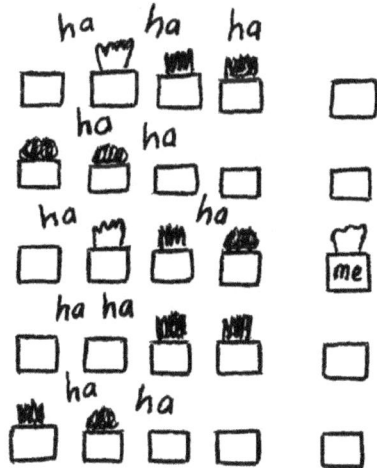

Girls and Guys

- I find it so much easier to talk with guys than girls.
- I like to talk about information and technical topics and learn new stuff.
- As a kid, I liked riding motorbikes, climbing trees, and building cubby houses. I didn't like dolls or playing house.
- I don't like to talk about superficial things, but to talk with intensity.
- I don't behave like a neurotypical woman. I get on better with guys, probably because I am information-based, and I can joke and banter with them. Women are more likely to follow 'social rules' and when I don't follow those rules I can be rejected.
- I remember a group of girls crowding around a mum with a new baby. They were asking how she and the baby were and saying how lovely the baby was.
- Then I came in with a technical question, 'Are you using cloth nappies or disposable?'
- The girls all stopped looking at the baby and stared at me.

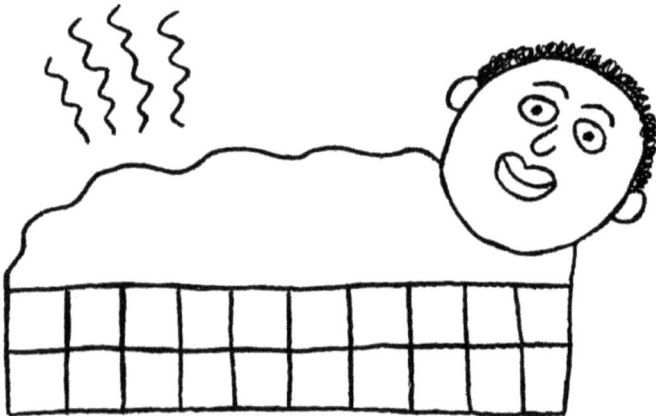

Instinct

- I seem to act on instinct, helping people and then realising maybe I shouldn't be there. I feel it is my responsibility to help because no one else is.

- Once when travelling in Italy, I saw a little old lady clinging to a wall struggling to get down a very steep path. I went to her, put my arm out and led her down the long path (no words were spoken). She was so grateful, bowing and bowing.

- I was so worried about Oliver because I was gone for a while, and he would not know where I was.

- Another time my job entailed that I took the banking to the bank. On the way back to the office I saw an old lady struggling with her shopping. I carried her shopping back to her unit and helped put her groceries inside.

- I was very worried that if my employer found out where I was, I would be in big trouble.

- The last story is when I lived with two flatmates (one girl and one guy). The guy tried to kill himself several times. Once he gassed himself in his car, but the police found him just in time. He was placed into a mental hospital.

- My other flatmate and I visited him in the hospital. His whole family gave up on him.

- The psychiatrist called us in to give his report on our flatmate – this was so weird because we had only known this guy for a short time.

- The other flatmate stopped visiting but I kept going; he had no one else.

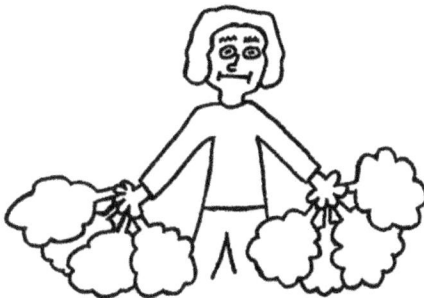

Bloody Tea

- Age: early 30s
- I didn't know that you offer people a drink when they visit you in your house.
- My friend visited me, and I sat at the table waiting for her to tell me her news - why else would she be visiting?
- After a bit of waiting she jumped up, stormed into the kitchen, and said, 'I'll make my own bloody tea then.'
- I thought, 'Yeh, OK,' but I didn't help her as she tried to find the cups, teaspoons and teabags.
- I could see her in the kitchen from my place at the table, and I thought it was a great game to watch her get more and more annoyed when she couldn't find things.
- When the game was over and she had found everything, she offered me a cup of tea.
- What a great visitor/host she was.

Reading Faces:
What I thought
my friend was thinking:

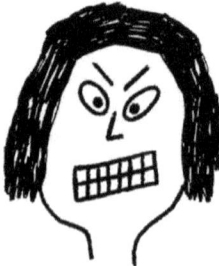

A. Why isn't Virg making the bloody tea?
B. This game is hard
C. Ow, period cramp

No, not there, keep looking, this is so funny, no, not there either

Answer:
At the time, I thought it was B.
The answer is probably A.

Taboo Shops

- Age: late 40s
- At some shops, my black and white, love and hate brain kicks in.
- One time was at a chemist where the shelf tags advertised that if you bought a product, you would get an extra item. I bought that product and went to the counter to get my extra item. The cashier/manager said, 'Sorry we've run out.' I said, 'Well why is the advertisement still on the shelf, can I have another item?'
- She looked at me, snorted and said, 'Of course not.' I wanted to rip the tags off the shelves and not buy the products, but we needed them, and we were in a hurry. So, I bought them, but afterwards I boycotted that chemist for years.
- Another time was at an antique shop. I was curious where the manager got her stock from and asked which auction she attended. She told me the days the auction was on.
- When we left the shop, Oliver said she sounded like she was making up answers; he got a bad feeling from her and told me she was lying.
- So, both these shops are now 'Taboo Shops'. We can't visit them again if the people managing them are liars and cheats.

Taboo shops

- chemist ✗
- antiques ✗
- pets ✓
- shoes ✗
- furniture ✓
- books ✓✓
- chocolate ✓✓

'SOME PEOPLE GET ANGRY WITH ME'

10

WHAT DO I DO?

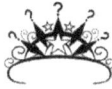

- Not for Me
- How Much
- Car Crash
- Haircut
- Indoor Cricket
- I Believe You
- Clinking Glasses
- Stalking
- Yes or No
- Hello
- Questions
- Waiting
- Weather

Not for Me

- I remember in high school; the local roller-skating rink had a 24-hour skate.
- Some of my class went along and we met at the rink. Everyone put their bags down in one place and some people set up sleeping bags.
- For a few hours we all skated together.
- One time I was skating by myself and when I went back to my class, my bag was the only one there. Everyone else had moved somewhere else.
- I just stayed by myself and continued skating. I didn't know what to do.
- Another time, I was shopping and came across the coffee shop, where I saw about thirty parents from Aaron's class. Some recognised me and said 'Hi.' Others looked down, hiding their faces.
- I didn't hang out in the carpark after school gossiping with the other adults. I enjoyed being with Aaron at school and went to the events I knew about, but I didn't do any extra socialising. I was invisible to the other parents.

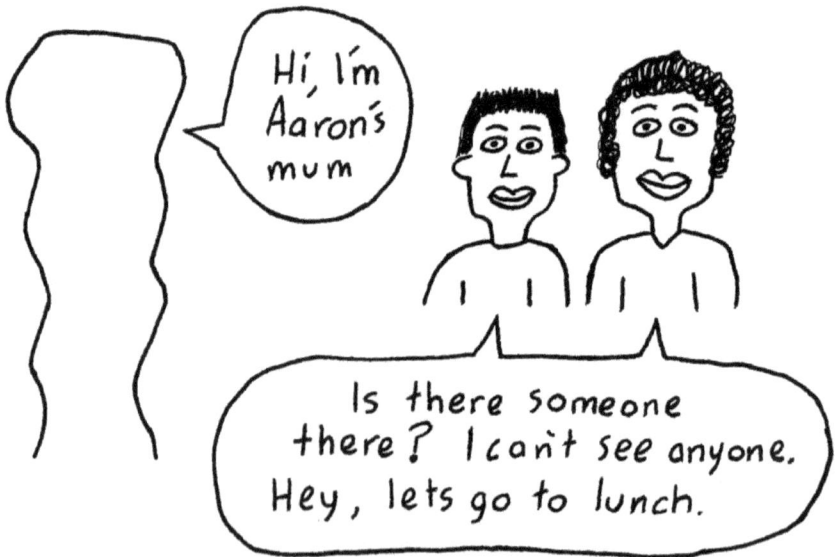

How Much

- 'How much' presents many different issues for me.

- I don't know when to stop - what information do I put in and what do I leave out?

- In high school, I had to do a timeline assignment. The teacher showed the class another student's assignment, one page. Then he showed mine. He stood on a chair and held my assignment up. The pages went to the floor and across the room for metres. I remember I got 19 out of 20 - one point was taken off because I was a day late handing it in. It was late because the first draft wasn't neat enough for me and so I tore it up and re-wrote and re-drew the entire thing.

- When I talk to people, I tell them everything. I go right back to the beginning, giving history and all the details and finally to my current story. I just don't know how much information to say.

- If I start a story, I want to give the whole story, I don't want to stop halfway. I want to keep talking. It is painful for me to stop.

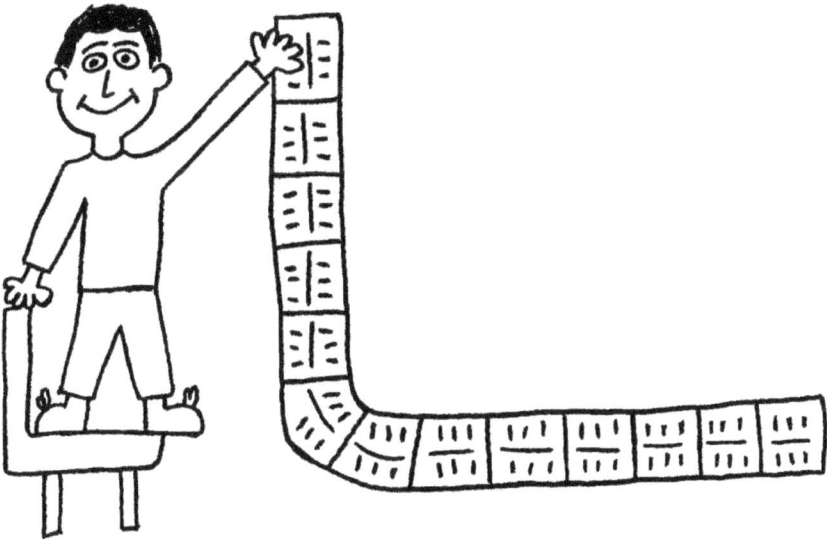

Car Crash

- Age: early 20s
- My friends and I were at a nightclub. I was the designated driver.
- When we walked back to my car, there were police and fire trucks with lights flashing right near my car.
- I saw my car and it was written off, totally smashed.
- Someone had sped down the road and hit my car (first in the row), which hit the car behind. Nine cars in the line were damaged.
- When I first saw my car, I was numb, I didn't really have any emotion, I just felt blank.
- Then I saw that my friends were really upset, so I ran to my car, threw myself on the bonnet and started screaming and thumping my arms, as I had learned from TV.

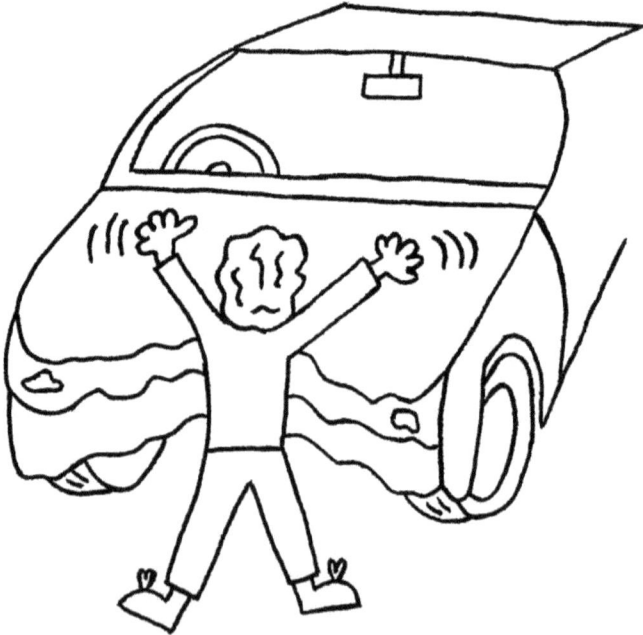

Haircut

- Age: early 20s
- A girl at work had a new haircut and to me it looked like she had been run over by a lawnmower.
- All the other girls in the office said her hair looked lovely. I thought they were lying to her.
- The office had about 20 staff and was quite open planned, just some pillars and short partition walls.
- I am no good at lying and was scared I would tell her that her haircut was really bad.
- For a long time, I hid from her, usually behind pillars. I was always on alert to where she was.
- Also, when someone was angry with me at work, I would hide from them for weeks until I saw them happy.
- The pillars became my best friends, we spent a lot of time together.

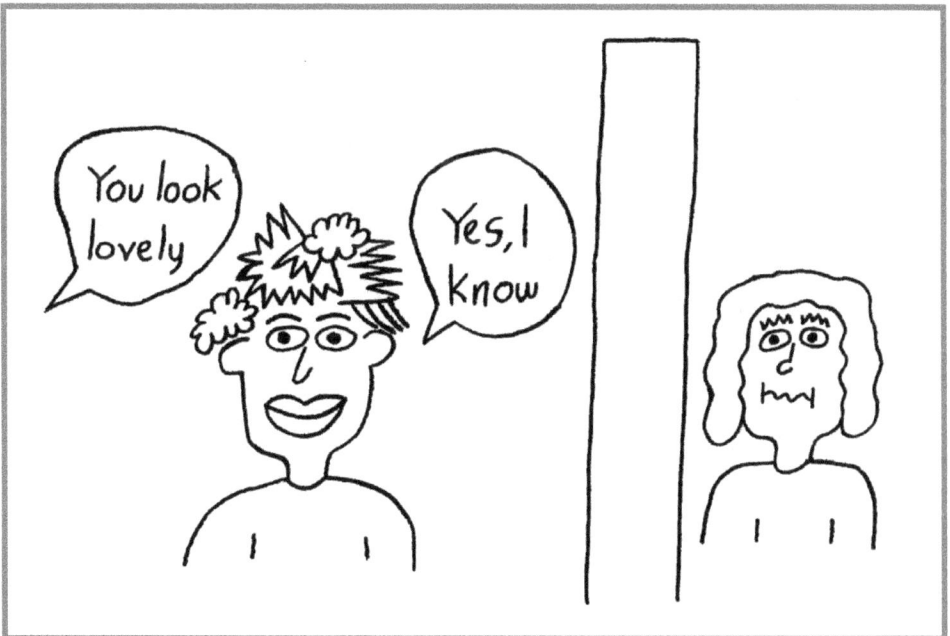

Indoor Cricket

- Age: early 20s
- I was playing indoor cricket. It was a mixed team, girls and guys.
- There was a gap in the fielding, so I stood there ready to catch the ball.
- A guy was batting, and he hit the ball really hard, right into my face (ahh, high school memories).
- I dropped to the ground, face down, and people crowded around me.
- I wasn't really worried about my face, but I started to panic about all the attention.
- I knew that on TV people screamed and yelled when an accident happened, so I started screaming and thrashing about, thumping my arms and legs, like a two-year-old having a tantrum.
- It worked because people started panicking.
- After the cricket accident, I went to the doctor. He gave me some drops and told me to live in the dark for a week. No scans or x rays were done.
- Thirty years later, after a face x-ray, I found out that I have been living with broken bones in my eye socket.
- Also, my eye has scarring and nerve damage, so I now need to take drops every night for eye pressure.

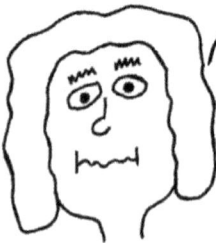

Thinking Back...
*I thought there was only one way to react.
I know now that I can stay calm in a crisis,
I don't need to overreact.*

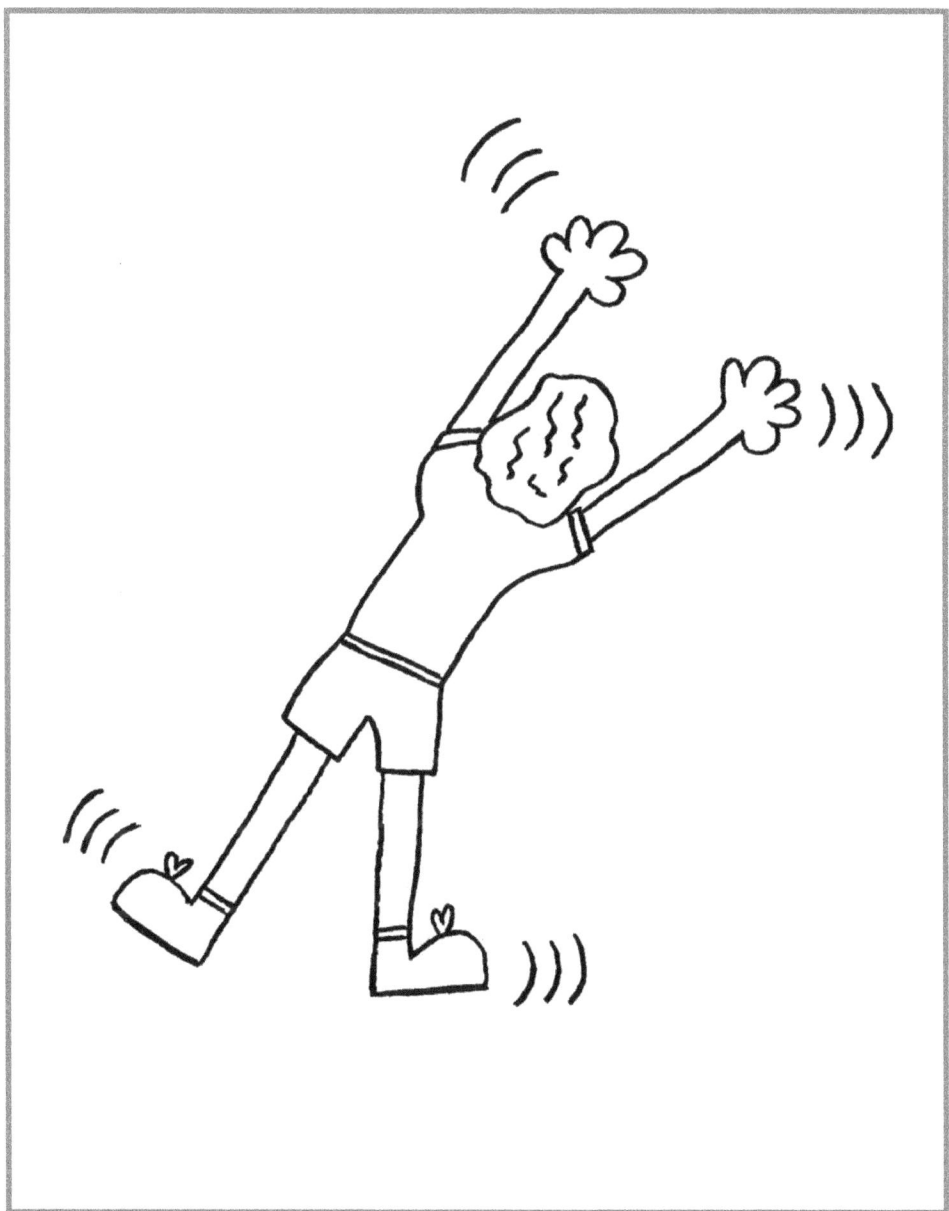

I Believe You

- A friend had a child the same age as Aaron.
- She suggested that we get together during the school holidays. She said, 'I'll call you and we will arrange something.'
- I waited at home for the whole two weeks, waiting for her call (mobiles didn't exist back then). I didn't go out, I just stayed home waiting for the phone to ring.
- She never called.
- I then broke up the friendship.
- Some people said to me, 'Why didn't you call her?' Well, she said she would call me, not the other way around.

silence

MAY
M T W T F S S
1 2 3 4
5 6 7 8 9 10 11
12 13 14 15 16 17 18
19 20 21 22 23 24 25
26 27 28 29 30 31

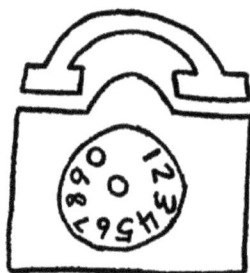

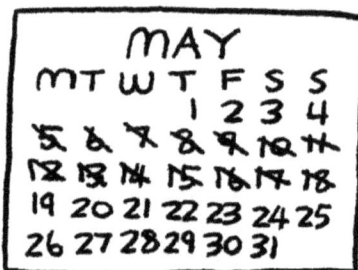

← phones before mobiles

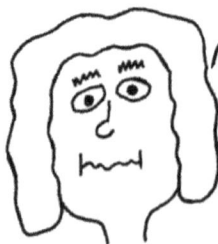

Thinking Back...
I know now that people say things just to be nice, and that I shouldn't believe everything I hear.

Clinking Glasses

- Age: early 40s
- At a dinner in a restaurant, we were celebrating someone's birthday and clinking glasses of drink together, 'Cheers'.
- One person was clinking glasses all around me but didn't touch my glass.
- I straight away thought I must have done something to upset her.
- I spent the rest of the dinner worrying, trying to rack my brain with what I had done in the past to upset this person.
- It must be me, I've done something wrong.

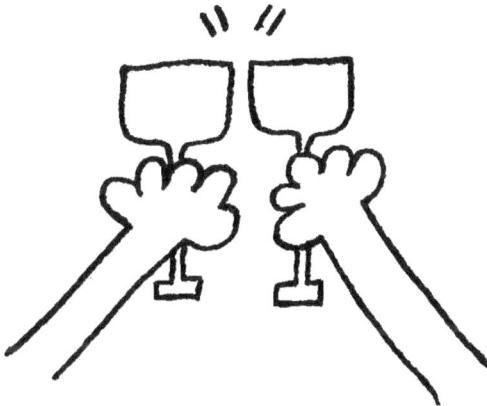

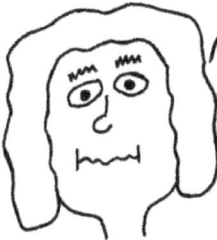

Thinking Back...
There is nothing in this, the person just accidentally missed my glass. It is not a strict procedure where the world will blow up if someone's glass doesn't get clinked.

Stalking

- When I worked at a supermarket, there was one lady who paid a lot of attention to me.
- I would tell her everything, 'spill my guts'. Every time I worked with her, I would hunt her down and tell her more. It was like free counselling.
- At other times when I have been talking with someone and they leave the room, I will follow them and keep talking. When they stop and sit down, I sit down next to them and continue.
- I do finally get the message when we have moved to several different locations and the speed of the pursuit has increased.
- I realise now this is called 'stalking'.

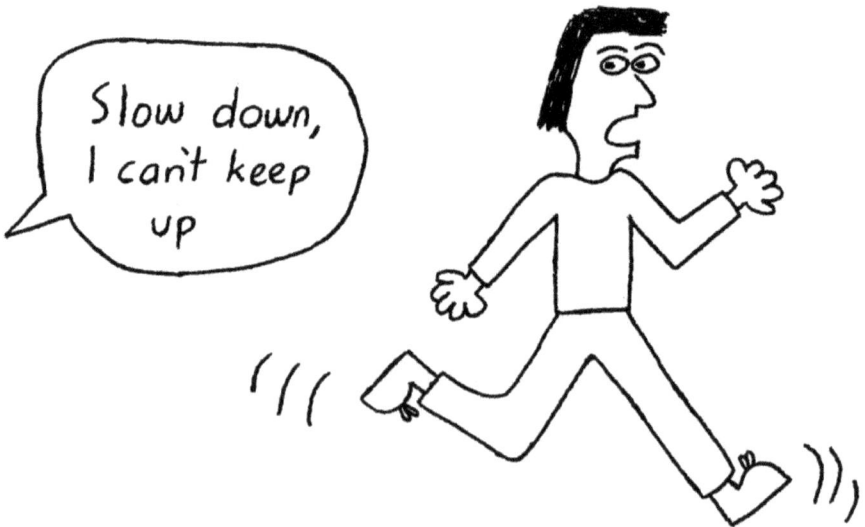

Yes or No

- Many times, people want a 'Yes' or 'No' answer. I try to answer 'Yes' or 'No', but I can't. They think I am being annoying on purpose but to me it just isn't that easy to answer 'Yes' or 'No' e.g., 'Would you like an ice cream?' Well what flavour, what size, is it creamy or a gelato, which shop will we be going to, are we going to buy anything else etc.

- One time I was asked, 'Are you growing your hair long?'

- I don't know, I don't have a hair schedule, hair just grows out of my scalp at the usual speed.

- Also, I remember one time when I forgot which way you move your head for 'Yes' or 'No'.

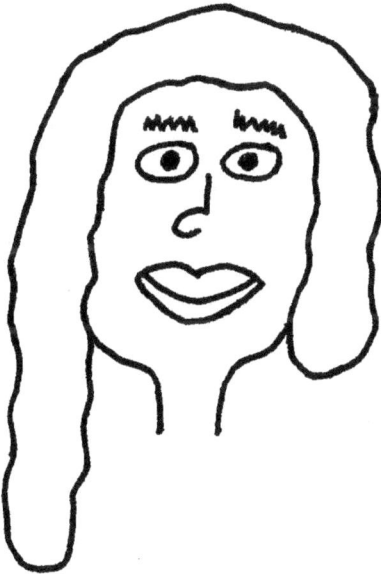

one side of my hair is growing long

Hello

- It is funny that people need you to say 'Hello' and 'Goodbye' every day when you are at work.
- If you don't, they make comments during the day such as, 'Well, hello, so nice to see you,' but I can hear from the tone that it is not nice to see me.
- One time when Oliver and I were shopping for electronics (we knew the person behind the counter), Oliver said, 'Hello' and then straight after he asked for what he wanted.
- I didn't know if I should still say 'Hello' because weren't we now past the 'Hello Time'?
- The person then said, 'Well, hello Virg.' I knew then that I got it wrong, 'Hello Time' doesn't end.

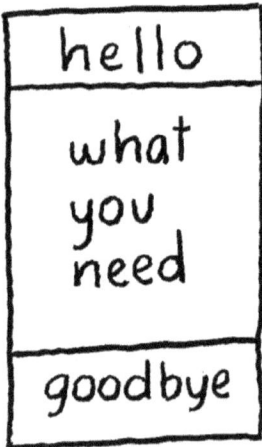

my way

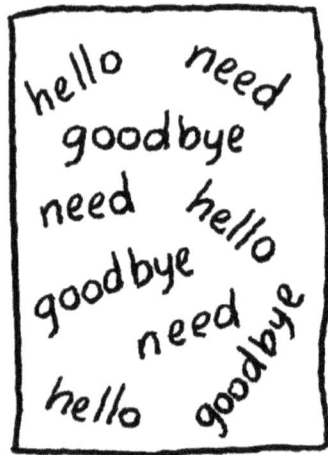

the other way

Questions

- There are a lot of interesting things about questions.

- I find people like to fire many questions at me. I try to keep up with them. I need to answer the questions in order. I don't just join the questions into one major answer.

- Some people get angry with me. They keep repeating the same question and I answer the same way each time. They think I can magically read their minds and come back with a different answer. Their voice gets angrier and angrier. If you want a different answer, ask a different question.

- Sometimes people ask the same question and I answer every question the same way, but this time they are not angry. Apparently, they are just reflecting on my first answer, and I don't have to keep answering.

- At times, when walking around, I hear strangers asking their friends questions, but no-one is answering them, so I answer them.

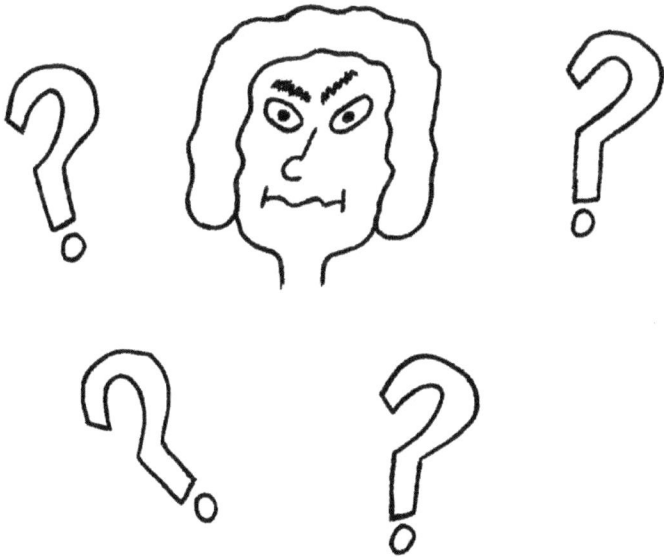

Waiting

- Age: early 50s
- Oliver, Aaron, and I went to a school reunion. Aaron and I were listening to another parent telling us about what his daughter was doing now.
- He then spotted someone and said, 'Oh, wait there, I just need to talk with _____ .' Aaron and I stood there wondering if we should really stand and wait or was that just social talking. We waited awhile and then walked off.
- Another situation was at a picnic. I was talking to someone, and she suggested I talk with _____ about massage (I didn't really know this person). I went over to _____ , who was making her lunch, and she said, 'Just wait, I'll just finish this.'
- I didn't know where to stand, thinking that if I was too far away she would forget about me, too close and it is stalking. So, I stood nearby, but I was really worried my distance was not correct.

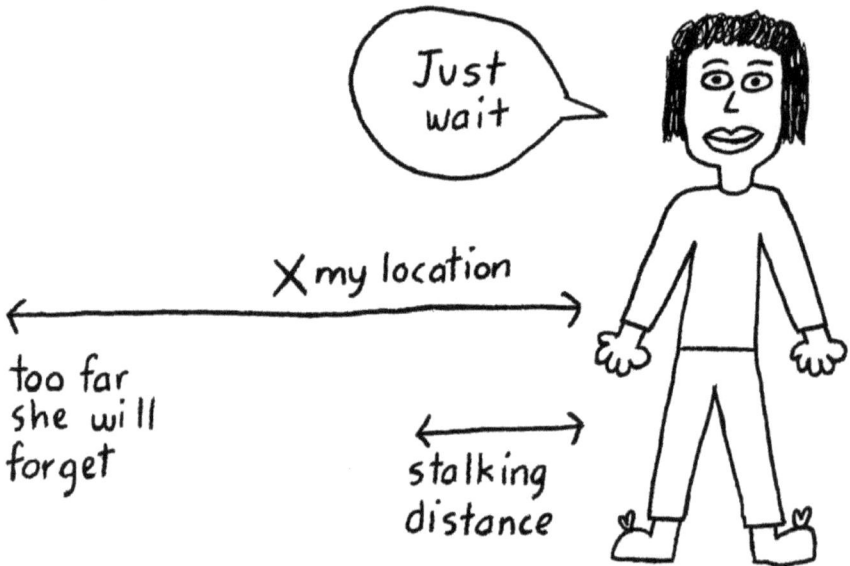

Weather

- Age: early 50s
- People and psychologists would always tell me, 'Just talk about the weather.'
- I knew it was a common subject that everyone could talk about, but it always confused me because I had never heard people talk about wind speeds, air patterns or their favourite cloud formations.
- One day, Oliver was at his hairdresser, and I was sitting nearby.
- The hairdresser always talked about how hot or cold she was and how the temperature affected her.
- I was listening and then I had a major breakthrough. She was talking about the weather.
- All this time people had been talking about the weather, I never made the connection. To me the question should be, 'How does the temperature affect you?'

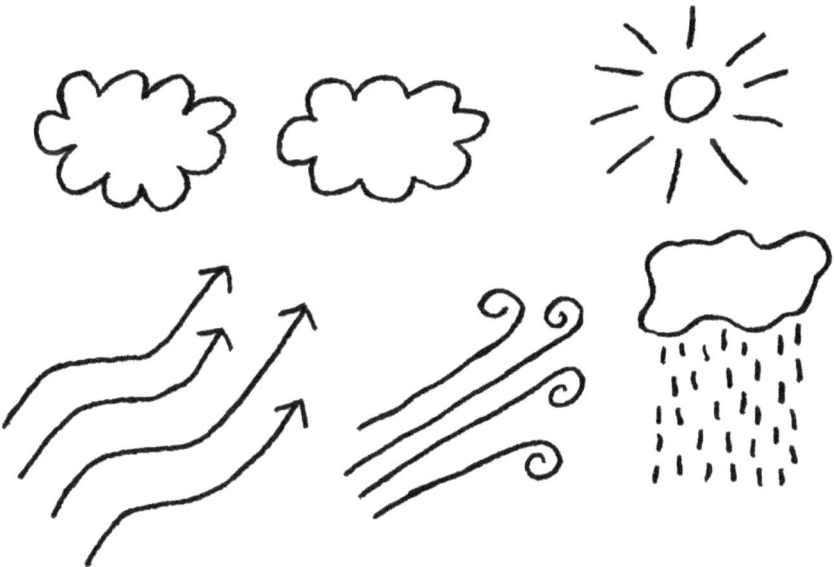

'IT LOOKED LIKE I WAS SOCIALISING'

11

SOCIALISING

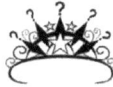

- Safe
- Dealing
- Socialising
- Superficial
- How Are You?
- Planning Social
- Conversation
- How to Greet
- Watching and Listening

Safe

- During my early socialising with Oliver's family (birthday parties and Christmas), I would sit with his mum and dad. There was no conversation, they just sat there, they didn't move around to socialise. I felt safe because I was always with someone; it looked like I was socialising.

- I didn't know how to join others in a group. Sitting or standing with a group has rules, different rules.

- We didn't know about Asperger's and Oliver just thought I was happy sitting there as he went to talk with his brothers and sisters.

- When Oliver's parents died, I was forced to get the courage to stand near people or sit in a spare seat. The more I did this, the more connections I made in my brain and the braver I got. My brain now had a formula.

- Also, when I meet people for the first time, I ask them many questions and tell them everything about myself. After meeting them for a few times, I have run out of questions and told them everything, things become difficult, what do I talk about?

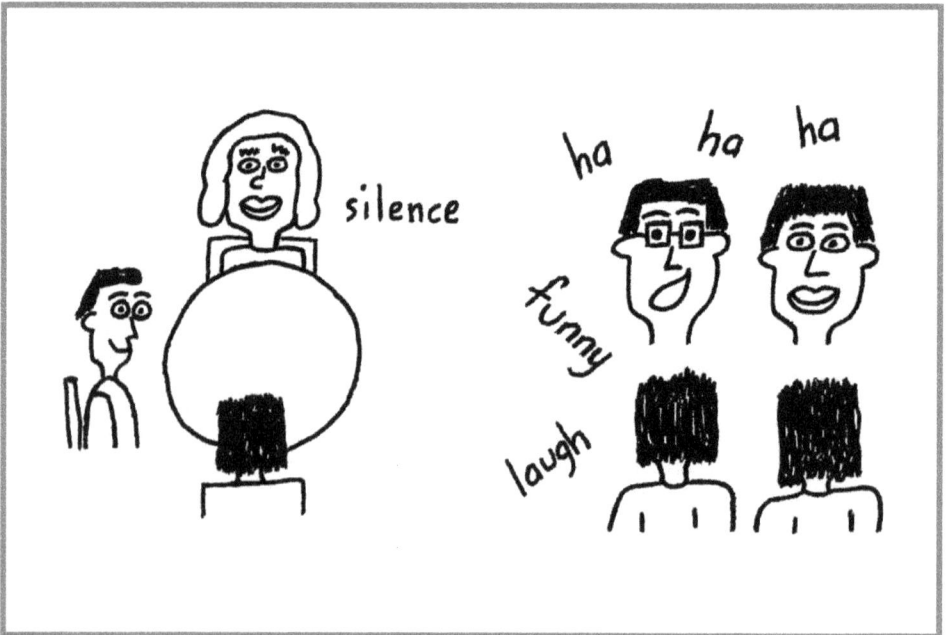

Dealing

- This is not a true story, but an example of how Oliver and I deal with problems. Let's say I lent someone a book and I want it back:

Me: 'Barry, you've had my book for one month, give it back.
You said you only needed it for a short while.'

Barry comes over and leaves the book on the front porch. The last two pages have been torn out and some of the other pages have strange brown marks on them. But who cares, I have my book back.

Oliver: 'Oh, hi Barry, how are you? How are Mary and the kids? Is Sammy still doing swimming? Oh, she won an award, well good on her. I'm fine, we're all doing well. Any holidays planned? Yeh, weather is looking good, great time to travel. Oh, yeh, we're planning a trip down south. Has Mary sorted out those eye issues she had? Did you watch the news, the weather in the eastern states. Yeh, I hope people are coping. Oh, I just wanted to check in with you, how you are going with the book I lent you?'

Barry: 'Oh, yeh, I was going to call you and drop it off today with some cake I made. I also wanted to thank you so much, those last two pages on the 'Meaning of Life' and how to make more money than you could ever dream of, they changed my life. I made so much money that I wanted to give you a bag of cash along with the book and the cake.'

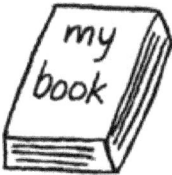

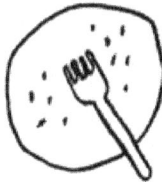

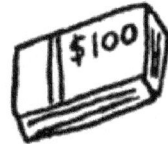

Socialising: Oliver vs. Me

Oliver and I have different socialising methods.

OLIVER	ME
• Oliver pretends to pay attention to people when they are talking to him. Afterwards I ask him what they said. He answers, 'I don't know, I wasn't listening.'	I remember and retain what people tell me, and after some time remind them what they said. Then they get angry and say, 'No, I didn't say that.' They don't have my memory skills.
• Oliver ignores bossy people.	I get hooked in by bossy people. I don't want to, but I believe I must pay attention to them.
• Oliver says, 'I'll call you' or 'I'll have to lend you that book.'	I ask him afterwards if he called them or dropped off the book. He says, 'No.' I start panicking.
• Oliver is too polite to laugh.	I laugh at what I think is funny, only to have people get angry with me.
• Oliver says to me, 'Yeh, I'll do that later.'	Later is not a time. I want to know when.
• Oliver makes the same mistakes over and over.	I remember how past events went. If you do 'this and this' it will end like 'this'. There is usually a pattern.

Superficial

- Age: late 30s
- I was planning a four-month trip to the northern part of Western Australia.
- At a business/friend get-together, someone asked me, 'How is your trip planning going?'
- I went into a two-hour answer giving all the information, my research, my notes, all the details.
- She then gave me an angry face.
- I thought, 'Oh, she is jealous,' and I continued with my very important information, smiling to myself thinking, 'Ha, ha, you're not travelling.'
- She says 'Oh, there is _____ , I'm going.'
- At home, I replayed the event to Oliver. I was worried that she seemed angry.
- Oliver explained that she only wanted a superficial answer.
- I had never heard this word before and when Oliver tried to explain 'superficial' to me, I sobbed and sobbed. Why had no one ever told me this before?

Reading Faces:
What I thought
she was thinking:

A. I'm so jealous!
B. I've got a headache.
C. When is she going to shut up?

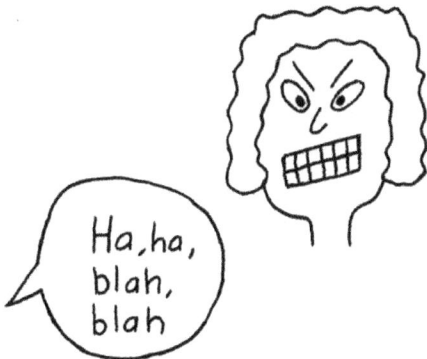

Ha,ha, blah, blah

Answer:
At the time, I thought it was A.
The answer is probably C.

How Are You?

- Age: early 40s

- Oliver taught me that when someone asks me, 'How are you?' I was to say 'Good' and ask them, 'How are you?' back.

- I thought I would try this at a picnic. There was a friend visiting from Singapore.

- She asked, 'How are you?' I answered 'Good,' and added, 'How are you?'

- She answered, 'Blah, blah, Singapore, blah, blah, waffle, waffle, shopping, blah, blah, food, blah, blah, waffle, waffle.'

- I asked a relevant question: 'What is the population of Singapore?'

- She made a constipated face and continued waffling on.

- Next, she sees someone and states, 'Oh, there is _____ , I'll just go say Hi,' and she leaves me sitting alone.

- I thought, 'This asking 'How are you?' is crap. I have to listen to people waffle on, I don't get a turn, then I'm sitting alone, and I don't know the population of Singapore.'

- I won't do that again.

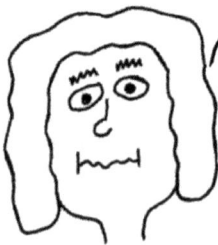

Thinking Back...
People like to waffle on, they don't usually want to talk about facts.

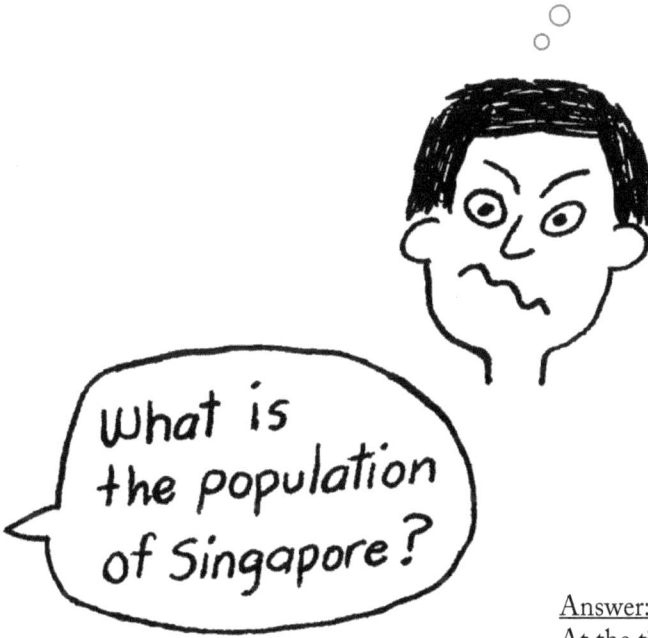

121

Planning Social

- When it comes to social, I need time to make plans in my head. It is very stressful to be told to socialise tonight, without warning.
- I like to practice answers and questions to an imaginary social event, so that I am prepared for the real thing. Of course, the socialising never works the way I practised it.
- I worry days before and will use my 'Superpowers' to try to have the event cancelled.
- I want to arrive on time because there are less people to greet and I can find a place to stand or sit.

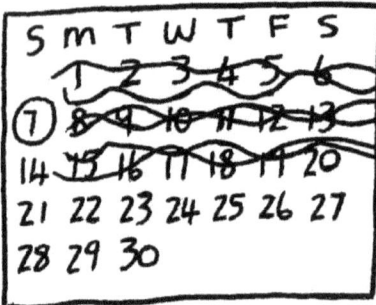

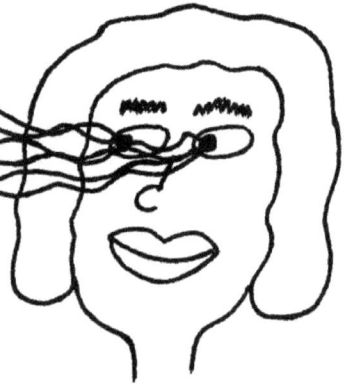

using my 'Superpowers'

Conversation

- How I have a one-on-one conversation at a party:

  1. First, I stress for days about the upcoming social event, planning questions in my head and then practicing them.
  2. At the event, I begin talking with someone.
  3. I start noticing how my mouth is moving and then the movements become weird, exaggerated. My eye starts twitching.
  4. Soon I am producing excess saliva and spit is flying out of my mouth.
  5. I ask myself, 'Have I looked into the eyes enough, was that too long?'
  6. More questioning myself. 'Am I still on topic? Was that a question, do I need to answer that?'
  7. Ah, too much silence, must fill the silence.
  8. Oh, I'm talking too fast and loudly.
  9. Then my beer-holding hand starts shaking. The person looks at this and probably thinks, 'Is she drunk?'

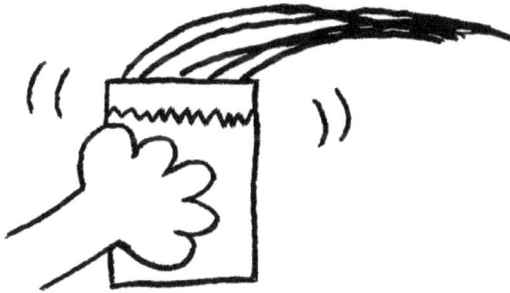

- Note: if I don't have a drink in my hand, I like to hold a rolled-up serviette and move it around in my hands for stress relief.

How to Greet

- Greeting people can be very difficult. At times I can go in for the peck on the cheek and find myself head-butting the person or poking them in the eye.
- Oliver and I were involved in a church choir. Oliver would say 'Hi' and kiss everyone and sit down. I would hug them, rub their backs, kiss, and then take ages to say 'Hi' to everyone. Oliver would be sitting there watching me take forever.
- I asked him how come he was so fast. He explained his technique. He would put one hand on their shoulder, lean in and 'peck a kiss and leave'. I practiced the technique and it worked.
- On other occasions, I would wait and see what the other person did and copy them e.g., reach a hand out for a handshake or hold both arms out for a hug or just say 'Hi' with no arms, meaning no touching.

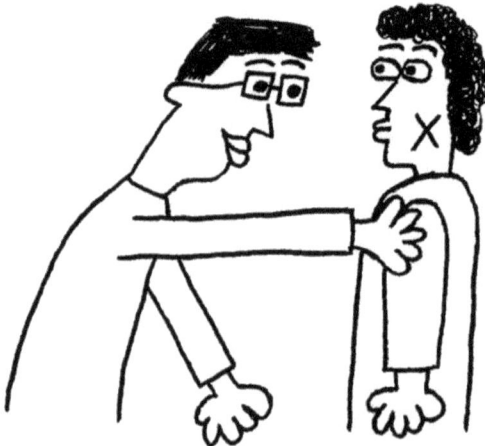

Oliver's technique

Watching and Listening

- I have spent my life watching and listening to other people.

- I stand close enough to listen but camouflage myself by doing an activity. I am not listening so that I can then spread information, it's just my way of learning social without the stress of socialising.

- There was a group of people Oliver and I spent time with. There was always dinner at a table involved. One person needed a lot of attention and would stand up and tell bad taste jokes or push her point of view. I would watch her and notice the negative response from the other people. She taught me a lot on what not to do.

- Something I worked out for myself: be a talker not a blabber. When I am a blabber, I tell too much from my heart and worry later about what I said. When I am a talker, I don't invest any of my heart, I speak superficial, empty talk.

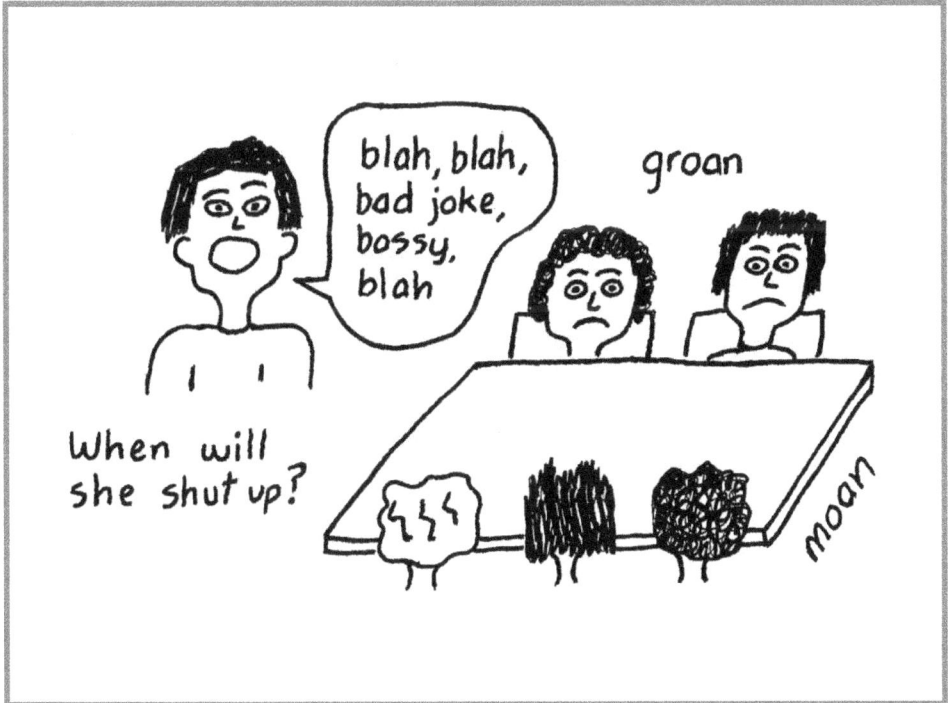

'1 AM BRUTALLY HONEST'

12

RULES AND LYING

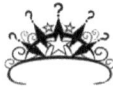

- Adult Rule Book
- Rules Rule
- Lying Rules
- Social Rules
- Are They Lying?
- Hiding a White Lie

Adult Rule Book

- I have a childlike way about me.
- The story in my head is that I didn't get the 'Adult Rule Book'.
- I like to use my emotions fully e.g., if I am angry, I'll show anger.
- I get super excited about small things e.g., patterns and pictures on a cup.
- I can come across as immature and naïve.
- Others can tease me, and I don't realise that this is what they are doing until someone else tells them to stop.
- I assume that people are good, and when I find they are not behaving nicely, it really upsets me. I just don't understand why they act that way.
- I am not afraid to ask any questions, lots of questions.
- I have trouble getting my brain and mouth to work together and I can sound childlike.
- I am brutally honest and tell people their errors.
- I still get quite emotional, and I will cry if I see bullying.
- What you see is what you get with me.

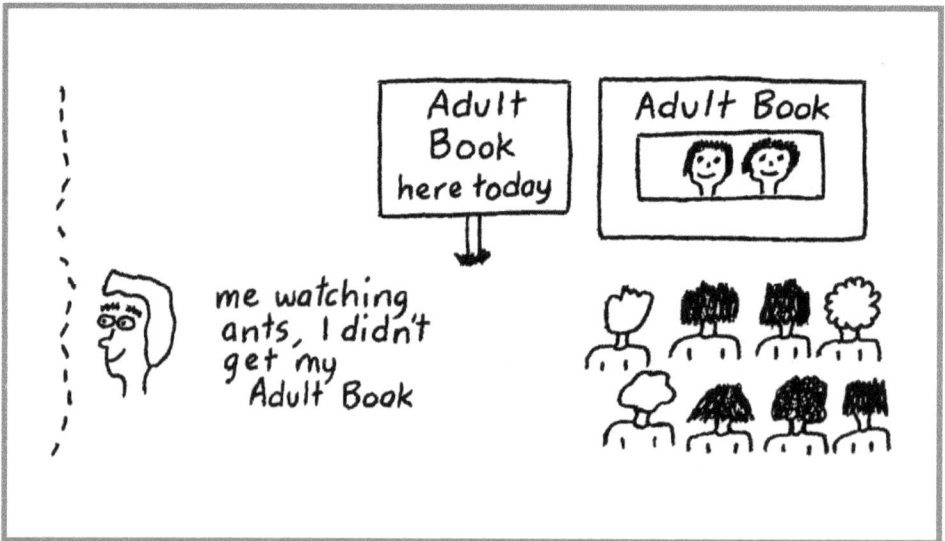

Adult Book here today

Adult Book

me watching ants, I didn't get my Adult Book

Rules Rule

- For me, rules are not set to annoy, but to keep people safe. For example, we wanted to take photos inside a historic swimming pool in Melbourne. We asked and were told 'No, because of privacy issues.' It made sense, not everyone likes photos of themselves in bathers or maybe caught in the nude.

- I get really stressed if safety rules aren't followed.

- I follow rules even if it disadvantages me. Oliver says, 'Why are you doing that to yourself, putting yourself through all that pain?'

- When Oliver doesn't obey rules, Aaron and I tell him off.

- We feel rules help keep order and people safe. Rules give us a feeling of oneness and love.

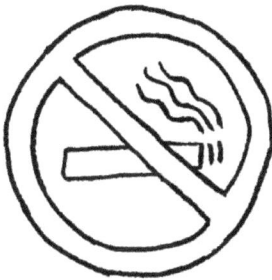

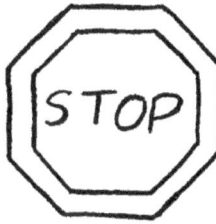

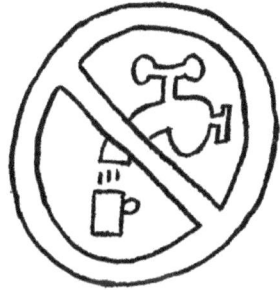

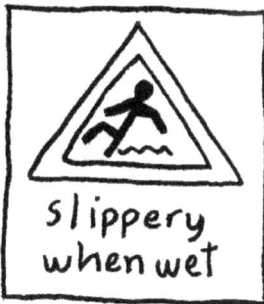

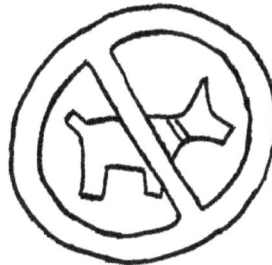

Lying Rules

- I find lying hard. There are so many components to a lie, how am I ever going to get them right? Sometimes neurotypical people just find themselves in a situation where they decide to tell a lie because it seems easier than trying to explain everything, but this is difficult for me.

- For example, Oliver and I once booked into a training camp, but at the last minute another opportunity came up and Oliver decided to go to that instead, leaving me to explain why he wasn't with me. I tried to make up a story, but I know I gave too much information, my voice went all weird, I couldn't look at anyone and I was edgy and jumpy. Much later I gave even more information to help back up my lie.

- How to show that you are lying:

  1. Use limited eye contact.
  2. Make sure your voice volume is not right – either too loud or too soft.
  3. Keep your body slightly skewed, not facing straight ahead.
  4. Set the tone of your voice in a higher pitch.
  5. Cross your arms – don't hold them in an open position.
  6. Exaggerate when you say things.

- People are so used to lying that when I say something that is true but strange, people cannot believe I am telling the truth. They say, 'Nah, you're lying.'

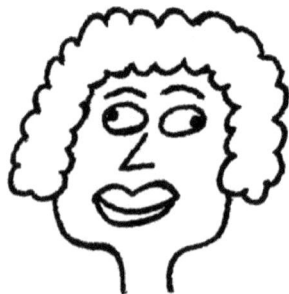

a liar

Social Rules

- I learned social rules from the television, not from my parents.
- Watching TV is easy. It is not social. There is no human connection and I can just watch and learn and not get caught out staring.
- I follow social rules such as 'RSVP'.
- If I need to RSVP or I can't attend, I will phone.
- If an invitation says 'Bring a plate', I will always do that.
- When people tell me, 'Don't tell anyone what I told you,' I don't, but it is very confusing when I see them telling others the forbidden information.
- I always use manners like thank you, please and excuse me. Manners make people feel good and then they will be nice to others.

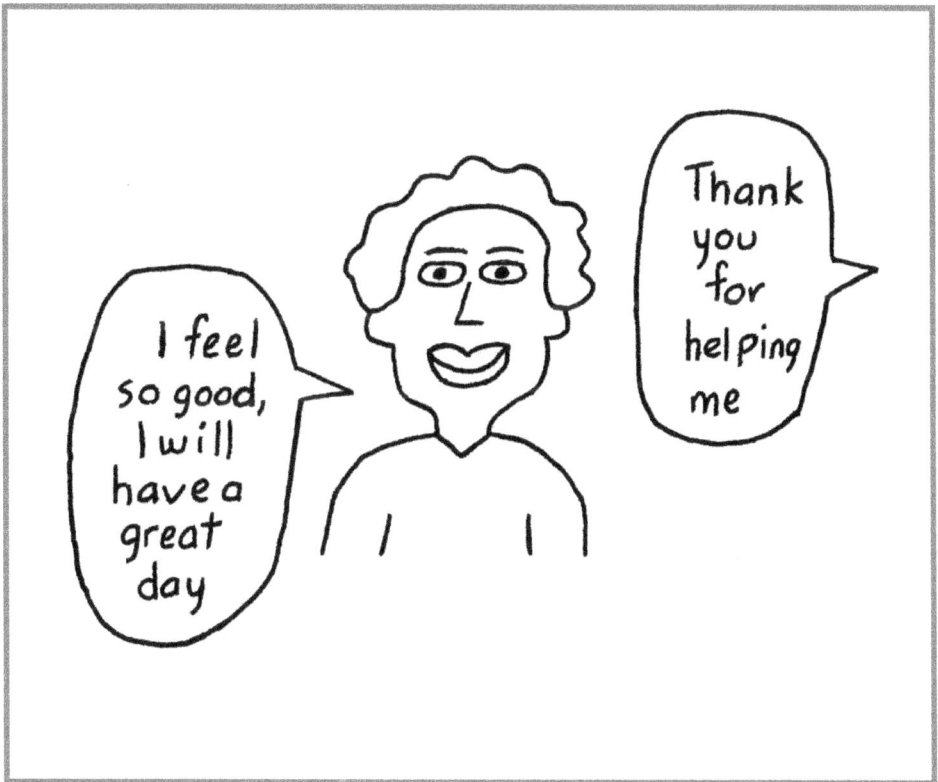

Are They Lying?

- I don't like people who are dishonest or manipulative.
- I want to expose them, let them know that I see what they are up to.
- I don't trust liars or manipulators. I know they are operating from a hidden agenda. They are misleading people for their own benefit.
- At times, I believe people are hurting me on purpose. They are manipulating me.
- I also believe that if people say they don't remember something, they are lying.

Daily Energy and Emotional meter - each dash equals one hour, don't waste your day	Good Day - watching TV - time with Aaron - play with dogs - eating food - Lego - fun with Oliver - exercise - walk dogs - more Lego - read books	Bad Day - telling off liars - fighting - crying - worrying about past - correcting people - reviewing day - errors made - screaming, shaking - TV, Oliver, Aaron - Lego, dogs

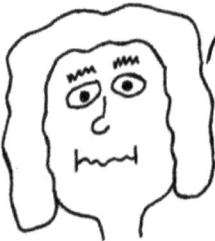

Thinking Back...
I still get annoyed, but I just try to keep away from dishonest and manipulative people. Telling these people doesn't change them, I am just wasting precious emotions and energy.

Hiding a White Lie

- Let's say someone told Oliver and me that Mount Blah Blah was a great hike, and we should do it. We don't do it but we tell the person that we did, to make them feel like we appreciated their suggestion. Here is how Oliver and I would solve this type of problem:
- Person asks, 'How did you enjoy your hike up Mount Blah Blah?'

- Oliver:
- 'It was great, many steps. I liked it.'
- The End
- Oliver then has a relaxing time at home and sleeps peacefully.

- Me:
- I research Mount Blah Blah – count the number of steps, check out the view, the plant species, the time it takes to hike the mountain.
- I find photos from the internet and print them out.
- When I meet the person in question, I now have my answer ready. 'We climbed Mount Blah Blah on Tuesday 3 July. There were 372 steps. On the way we saw Bull Banksias and Lemon Honey Myrtles and the view from the top was over the fields to Mount Talk and the town of Liarville. It took us 5 hours and 23 minutes.'
- When the person pulls a funny face, I get up and block the door until they have seen my photo proofs (the internet pictures).
- Then I keep talking about how much I enjoyed the hike.
- Once they have left, I go over what I said and find the errors. Oh no - there were 369 steps and Lemon Honey Myrtles don't grow on Mount Blah Blah. They will know that I was lying.
- I have sleepless nights for months.
- I finally hike up Mount Blah Blah for real so I can get rid of some of the guilt for the lies.

'SMART PEOPLE ASK QUESTIONS'

13

LESSONS AND TRICKS

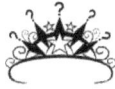

- I Know It, You Know It
- A Great Day
- Aaron Lessons
- People Patterns
- Lessons
- Matching
- Be Quiet
- Problems
- Tricks
- Boxing Ring

I Know It, You Know It

- We have a little Aspergian friend.
- When he was at our house, Oliver was making him a Milo (malted chocolate drink). Our friend came downstairs, saw Oliver making his Milo and had a mini meltdown, 'That's not how you make Milo,' scream, scream.
- I calmly and firmly told him, 'Have you ever told Uncle Oly how to make Milo before?'
- Our Aspergian friend calmed down.
- I added, 'Well go down there and tell him how to make the Milo.' He went over and told Oliver.
- Another time our Aspergian friend was mixing his Neapolitan ice cream into a brown sludge. Someone walked past and asked what flavour he had. He rudely stated, 'Neapolitan of course.'
- She said, 'Whatever, professor' and walked off. I said to our Aspergian friend that I only saw brown, I couldn't see any white or pink and I could not guess it was Neapolitan. He looked at his ice cream and understood.

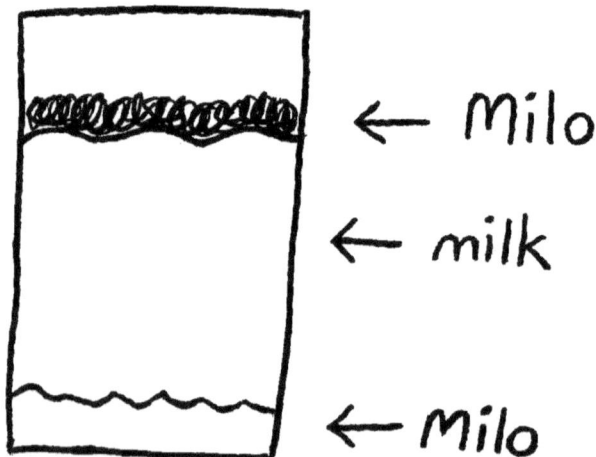

A Great Day

- We were looking after our little Aspergian friend. He had the day off school.
- We went shopping and he bought two small cars, then he got to choose a special lunch, go to two playgrounds, and play some computer games.
- In the afternoon, we went to do some food shopping and he wanted an ice cream. We said 'No' and he kept asking and receiving several 'Noes'.
- He became quite grumpy. I explained that he had had a great day with lots of good things happening, lots of 'Yeses'. I listed five things.
- He explained that today he had had more bad things happen than good things, five 'Yeses' and sixteen 'Noes'.
- I was a bit confused and asked about the sixteen 'Noes'. He said he asked for the ice cream sixteen times.
- I told him the rules: when you ask more than once for the same thing, it only counts for one thing.
- He accepted the rules and realised that he did get more 'Yeses' than 'Noes' and it was really a great day.
- He also got that ice cream.

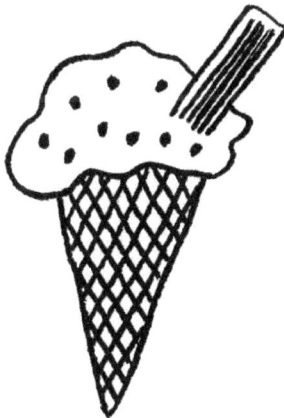

Yum

Aaron Lessons

- I learned a lot of useful tips in books and TV, things that made a lot of sense to me. Some things I worked out with my logical brain. Here are some:

- If your toddler complains during the night, give him/her a baby bottle of water and don't let them see your face. I filled Aaron's bottle with water and then commando crawled on the floor to his cot, raised my hand through the bars and gave him the bottle. He did not see my face. It worked.

- I gave Aaron warnings in a positive way, for example when your child is climbing a tree say, 'Hang on tight' not 'Don't fall.' The brain only notices the word 'fall'.

- I said 'No' to Aaron sometimes when I could have said 'Yes', just so he would learn to handle 'No'.

- When Aaron was naughty, I said to him 'It is not you, it is your behaviour which is naughty.' I remember a time when the dog chewed Aaron's soft toy and Aaron told him off using this technique.

- I always told Aaron to 'go through all the doors' (opportunities). He could always change his mind later, but we encouraged him to give anything a chance.

- Children like to know how far they can go, pushing boundaries (fences). They want the security of the 'fence' so they can bounce against it and back to a caring, secure person. Without it, they feel insecure. They want to know their limits.

- When giving compliments, be specific, e.g., 'That was a great goal you shot, straight through the middle,' not 'Great game.' It is an empty compliment.

- There are 'Yes' people and 'No' people. Some people just like to say 'No', keep searching until you find a 'Yes' person.

People Patterns

- I find that people follow patterns in the way that they behave.

- For example, when Aaron, who is a stable, happy, joking person, is quiet and agitated, I know he is not following his pattern, and something is bothering him.

- There are some patterns that are just the individual's, and then there is the 'common pattern'.

- A brilliant book about the 'common pattern' is *Personality Plus* by Florence Littauer.

- She explains about the four personality types, which I like to visualise to myself as a camping trip:

- 'Melancholy Personality' has the maps and details but worries about everything. 'Sanguine Personality' is excitable, just wants to get going but forgets her sleeping bag. 'Choleric Personality' organises everyone but can be bossy. 'Phlegmatic Personality' is loyal; you can depend on them, but they can be lazy.

- This book is so helpful to me. I can see which personality a person is, what pattern they are following, and I can understand why they behave as they do.

- I know 'Fake People' are acting, they are not being their genuine true self. They are not following the 'common pattern'. I can hear their tone is not normal and they don't act normal. I don't trust them; they are hiding something.

- There is also a pattern with what people do (not only how they behave). If people do 'this and this', then the outcome will be 'this'. The outcome is the same, it just has a different story leading up to it. People make the same mistakes over and over. I remember how past events went, if you do 'this and this' it will end like 'this'. There is a pattern.

Lessons

- These are some things I have learned along the way:
- Action cures depression.
- Everyone has good and bad in them.
- Smart people ask questions, dumb people think they know everything.
- If I am stressed, I bring myself into the 'Now' by feeling a part of my body like my feet on the ground, the clothes on my back, my tongue on my teeth.
- I have an internal meter. If Oliver is trying to help me with an issue, as soon as he says the right thing, I start crying. I know that is the answer. I fully trust my internal meter.
- The story of my past doesn't change, only the emotion I attach to the story.
- The more times I try something to do with socialising, the more connections I make in my brain. My brain now has a formula that it can repeat.

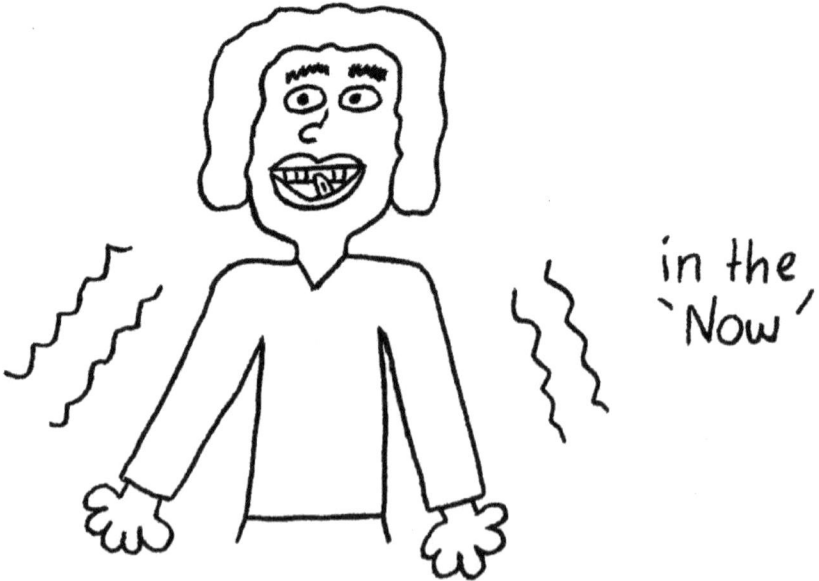

in the 'Now'

Matching

- When it comes to conversation, I find that matching topics works for me.
- If someone is talking about cats, I talk about cats or ask questions about cats.
- If I want to add some information about a past topic which was discussed, I say, 'Oh, when we were talking about dogs before, I forgot to say.' It works but only after a short delay of topic changes.
- If I know nothing about cats but I know about other types of pets, I can say, 'I don't know much about cats, but I love dogs.' I am still matching topics.
- I know not to talk and talk about the same topic because topic subjects change so fast.

topics to choose

Yes ✓	No ✗
· dogs	· Lego
· other pets	· reality shows
· beach	· clothes
· weather	· trains
· surfing	· farts
· swimming	· astrology
· sand castles	· football

I took my dog to the beach yesterday

Be Quiet

- Many times, I would tell people the truth, my truth.
- Often people would cry or be very angry and storm off.
- I didn't care about them; I just didn't like the friction, the tension I felt.
- Once a friend was showing Oliver their photos from a glamour/makeover shoot on the computer. I walked into the room and saw the photos from a distance. To me it looked like porn photos, and I almost said, 'Oh, who is the prostitute?'
- I looked more closely and saw who it was.
- I walked out of the room and started fist pumping. I was so proud of myself, and it felt so good to keep my mouth shut.
- If I feel like telling my truth again, I remember how good it felt to be quiet and not have the tension. It is a great and powerful feeling.

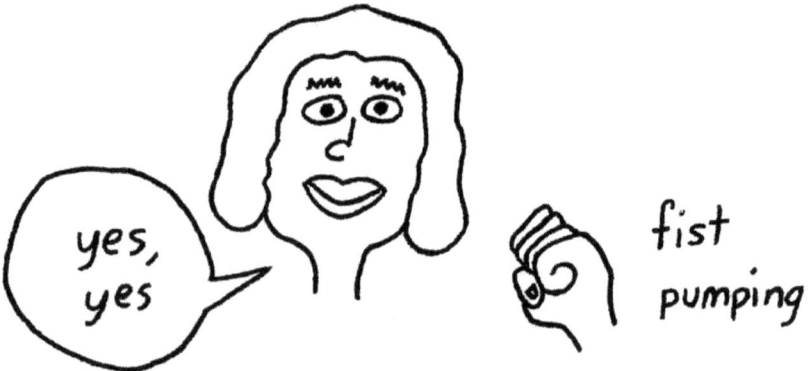

Problems

- Big problems and massive tasks are easy for me if they are not personal. Personal is when my heart is involved.

- With big problems, I take all emotions out and divide the problem into steps. Then I only work on the first step and wait until it is complete or someone else has completed the first step. If I go too many steps in front, it is wasted emotion, worrying about things that will probably not happen.

- When Oliver and I have our heart set on something and it doesn't work out, we find some other opportunity comes along that is better and we can see that the first opportunity would have hindered it.

- I use only logic to solve problems, there is no social involved. If someone proves by logic how to solve a problem, I will follow them with ease.

- Using logic and past experiences, I can solve problems fast. Often, if I tell a group of people the solution, they will ignore me. Oliver says they need to have the social interaction, people talking, tossing ideas around, feeling different decisions, analysing everything, feelings, feelings, feelings. If things are solved too fast, they believe it can't work. Often someone eventually comes up with my idea.

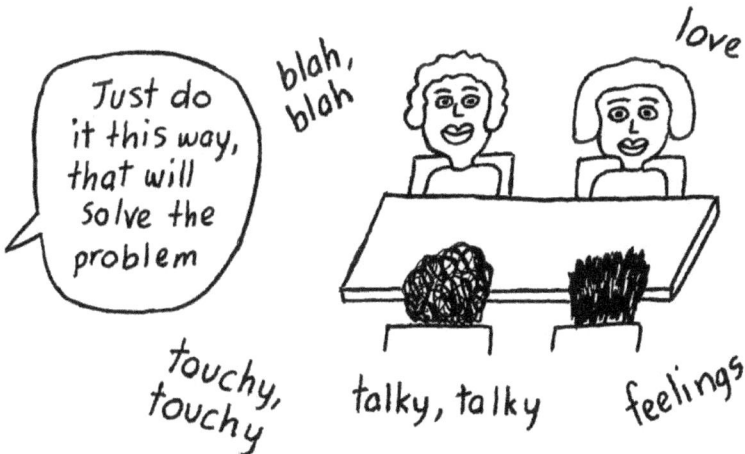

Tricks

- I have found some clever tricks to help me in life:

- I don't like flying on planes. I don't like the take-off, the landing, or the bit in the middle. The take-off is way too loud for me. So, I shut my eyes, put my fingers in my ears and pretend I am on a quad bike. I even rock sideways to really feel the motion. During turbulence, I do the same but imagine the quad bike is travelling over a very rocky section of track.

- Another technique is when I am sitting in a group, I don't have to say anything, just look in a direction where a conversation is happening.

- My humour can at times be a bit too much, so when I am talking and I see Oliver walk away, I know I have taken my joke too far.

- Another trick Oliver taught me: At a party, the DJ was asking for requests. I went to him and asked if he had a song I wanted. He answered, 'Yeh, yeh.' I waited and waited for my song. Twelve songs went by. I was angry, he lied to me. Oliver told me to use a number next time, say 'Five'. If I ask someone for any request and they haven't done it by 'Five', in this case five songs, it will probably not happen.

- When Oliver, Aaron and I were climbing a large mountain, there were really scary sections on the bare steep rock. There were white marks on the rocks to follow. I suggested to Aaron to imagine we were in a computer game and to gobble up all the dots. It worked; all our fear disappeared.

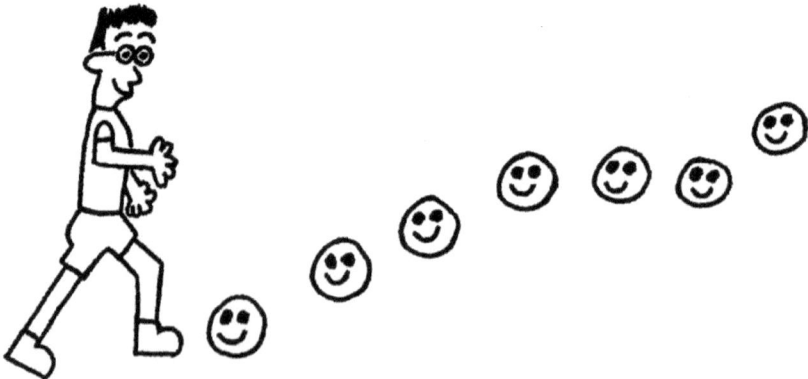

Boxing Ring

- I always had to get my point across to others, tell the truth and push and push my view. Or to tell people that they were lying or manipulating others.
- I didn't like the bad feelings and that some heated discussions didn't end until the other person had enough and walked away.
- It was so stressful and annoying. I didn't know how to stop the fighting. It wasn't that I cared about the other person's feelings, I just didn't like the feeling that I got.
- Oliver taught me a skill. If I didn't want to fight, then don't go into the 'Boxing Ring'. A heated discussion needs two people, if I don't enter the discussion (Boxing Ring) then there can't be a fight.
- When I tried this technique once or twice, it worked wonderfully. I felt so calm and peaceful which is so much better than pushing my view and feeling like crap.
- I just agree with the person (who wants to force his/her view) with no emotion.

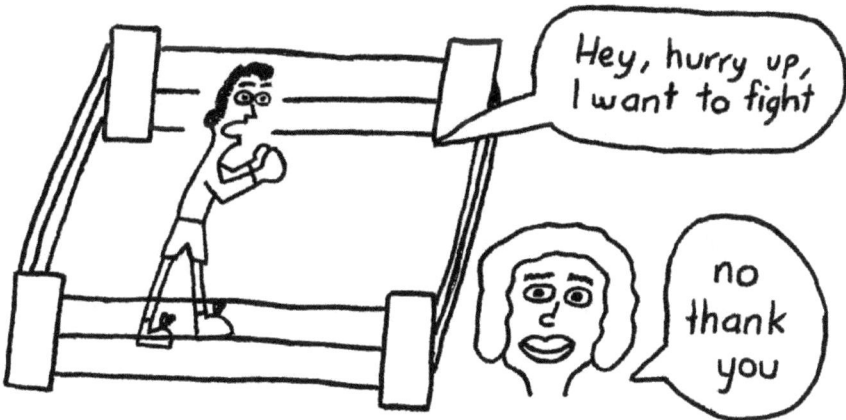

'SORRY GINA'

14

NOT WELL BEHAVED

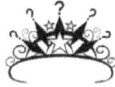

- Not Nice
- How Was Your Weekend?
- Not Dead Yet
- Gina
- Retirement
- Fun with Food

Not Nice

- There are many aspects of Aspergians that are not nice.
- To me correctness is more important than feelings. If a person is incorrect, I will keep pushing the correct way even if this upsets them.
- My worst trait is impatience. 'Now' is too late for me, 'Yesterday' is better.
- I interrupt conversations a lot. I just seem to get the gap in conversations wrong. People are just taking a breath; they have not stopped talking.
- I often ask inappropriate questions; I simply want to know information.
- I can also come across as boasting and bragging. I just get so excited with the things I do and want to tell people.
- I can be rude and arrogant.
- When people say they don't know, I believe that they are playing dumb or lying to me.
- I have been described as 'brutally honest'.

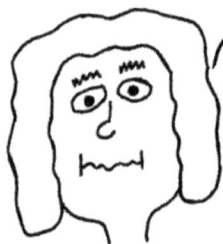

Thinking Back...
I have learned to keep my mouth shut.
When I keep my mouth shut,
my life is so much more peaceful.

How Was Your Weekend?

- Age: 20s
- At my workplace was a girl who always asked me, 'How was your weekend?'
- I knew that she only asked so she could then tell me about her weekend. I thought 'I know what you are doing, and I don't want to listen to your crap.'
- So, I would give an invented answer such as, 'Oh, I took my giraffe unicorn to London and visited the Queen.'
- Then I would walk away.

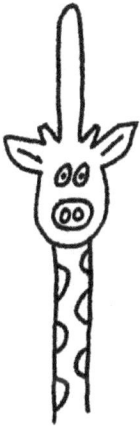

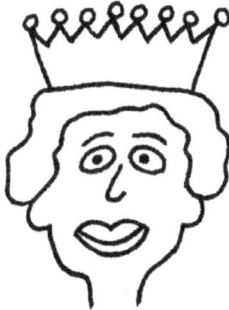

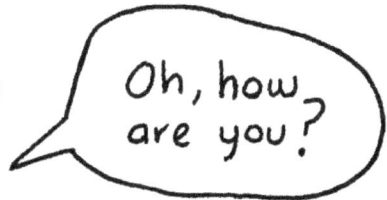

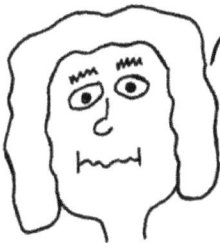

Oh, how are you?

Thinking Back...
I wasn't very nice at all.

Not Dead Yet

- Age: early 20s
- I believed that saying 'Bless you' after a person has sneezed originated from the time of the Great Plague when, if a person sneezed, they probably had the plague and were going to die. So, people offered a 'blessing' in the hope that they recovered.
- When people said, 'Bless you' to me after I sneezed, I would be annoyed and tell them, 'I just sneezed, I'm not going to die.'

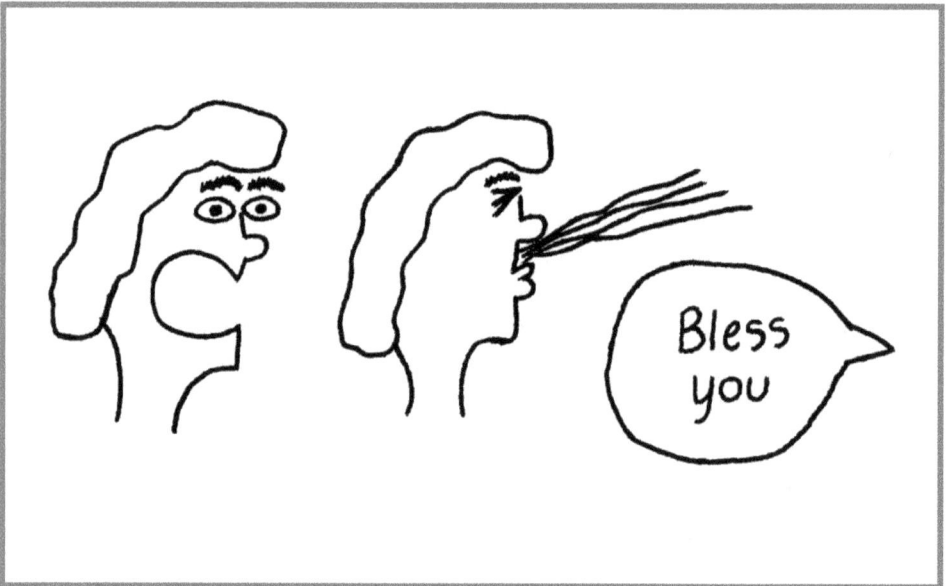

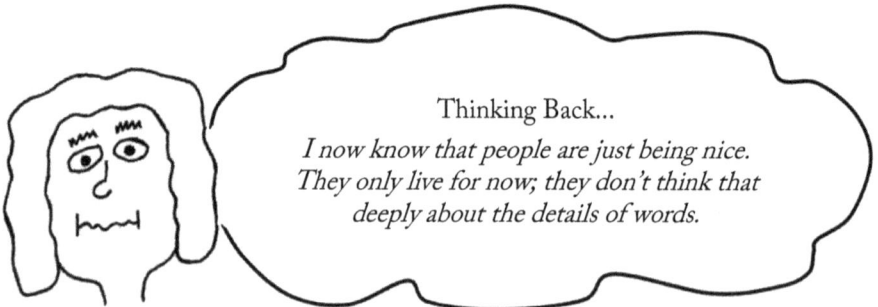

Thinking Back...
I now know that people are just being nice. They only live for now; they don't think that deeply about the details of words.

Gina

- Age: mid 20s
- When naming me, my mum liked the Dutch name 'Hena' which translated to 'Gina' in English. My mum didn't like the name 'Gina' so she made it longer and chose 'Virginia'.
- My dad called me 'Gina' along with other names.
- I hated the name 'Gina', it was not my name.
- A girl at one of the settlement offices I went to was named 'Gina'. We never spoke to each other but whenever I encountered her, I would give her evil eyes and an angry face. She would shrink and cower when she saw me coming. She probably thought I was a psycho. I hated her name so much that I made her scared of me.

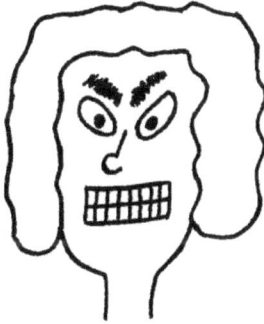

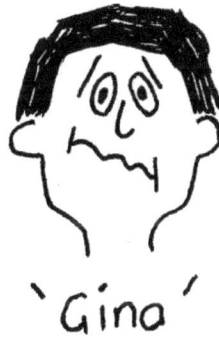

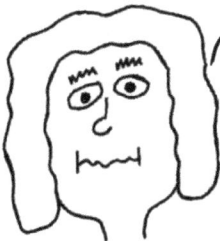

'Gina'

Thinking Back...
Sorry Gina.

Retirement

- Age: late 20s
- At one of my office jobs, a lady was retiring. All the staff had drinks after work for her farewell.
- She was asked what she would do in retirement. She said she was moving to a country town and had bought new furniture for her house including a new wardrobe.
- Next, she said, 'And then that will be it.'
- I thought that was so silly, she had retired and was now waiting for death.
- So I said, 'Oh, you can turn your wardrobe into a coffin.'
- Then all the attention went to the manager who was having a snorting/coughing fit and was running from the room.

retirement

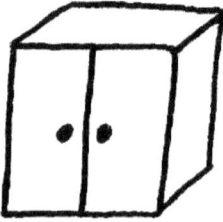
step one

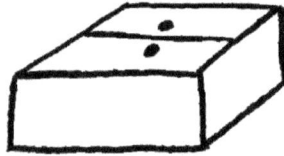
step two

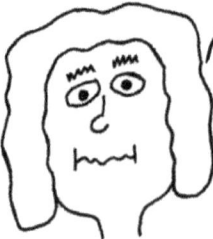

Thinking Back...
I now realise that the manager running from the room meant I went too far with my joke.

Fun with Food

- Age: late 30s
- At family get-togethers, there would be tables and tables of food, and we would all walk around with our plates, filling them up.
- There were some guys who I loved to 'joke' with.
- I would arrange food on my plate in a lovely pattern.
- I would then go up to my victim and say, 'Wow, the food here is great.'
- The person would look at my plate, then my face and back to my plate (I would keep my face very neutral).
- I could see them doubtfully thinking, 'No, it's just food, she wouldn't be naughty. I must not react, or I would look bad.'

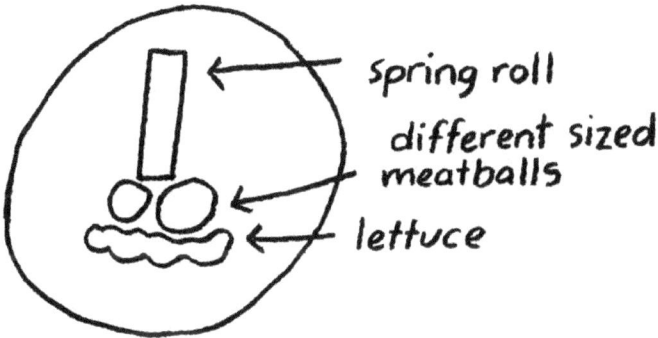

spring roll

different sized meatballs

lettuce

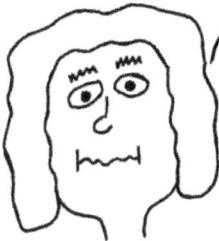

Thinking Back...
I was being naughty.
This is not something that should be copied.
It is not socially acceptable.

'LIKE IT IS PART OF MY SOUL'

15

SPECIAL THINGS

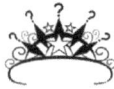

- Singing
- Collecting
- Details
- Reality Shows
- Stuff in Order
- What I Love

Singing

- I can sing pitch perfect.
- I have no musical training, but I have worked out what the notes on the sheet music mean, such as: length to hold the note, whether to move up or down the scale and the notes you sing together.
- I feel the music inside me like it is part of my soul. I just sing and emotion comes out.
- When I sing, I am nervous and shaking. I feel people can see inside me, I feel exposed.
- I have made people cry from emotion with my singing.

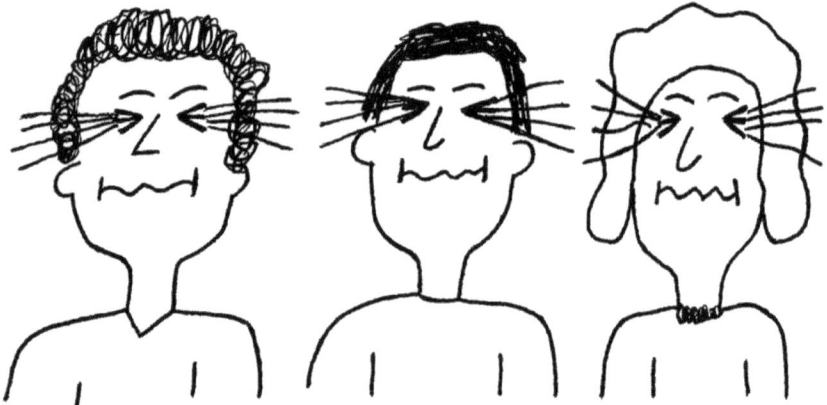

'I'm so glad you enjoyed my singing'

Collecting

- I love collecting certain things.
- Books:
  Young Adult - 421 books
  Australiana - 15 books
  Auto and biographies - 38 books
- Lego: 51 sets
- I only like Lego collector's sets such as Harry Potter, Simpsons, Minions, Flintstones, Beatles, Ghostbusters etc.
- Australian coins: 414 coins
- My books are in alphabetical order on my bookshelves.
- Lego sets are all in display cabinets.
- Coins are in folders in date order and are catalogued.
- At times I become obsessive and will spend time finding the missing items in the collection.

Interesting: the Australian Penny and Half Penny were made in Perth, Melbourne, Sydney, London, India, Sometimes in the same year, example 1951 Penny made in Melbourne, Perth and London

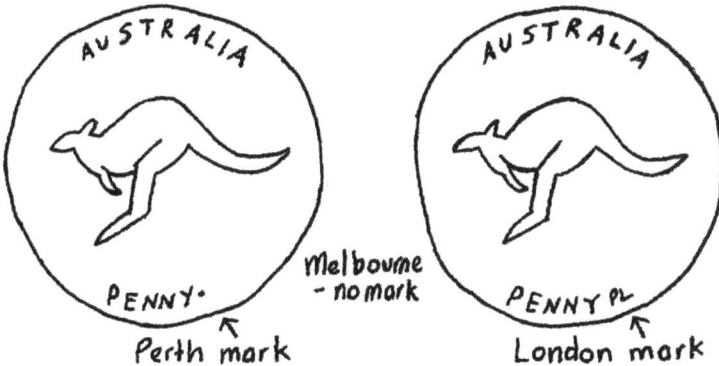

AUSTRALIA
PENNY·
Perth mark

Melbourne
- no mark

AUSTRALIA
PENNY PL
London mark

Details

- I have a very keen eye for details.

- Once I went to a church service and was looking at the enormous glass mural taking up the whole back wall. The mural had Jesus in the middle and abstract surrounds. It was made of many large glass panels. I noticed one glass panel had been put in backwards, the pattern did not match.

- When I go into a new room, I feel a mixture of anxiety and excitement. I like to find a gap and stand against the wall and then survey all the details in the room. I like to find the patterns.

- I take interesting photos of nature because I see the patterns in the rocks, plants, and trees. I get excited and point things out to Oliver, who didn't see them.

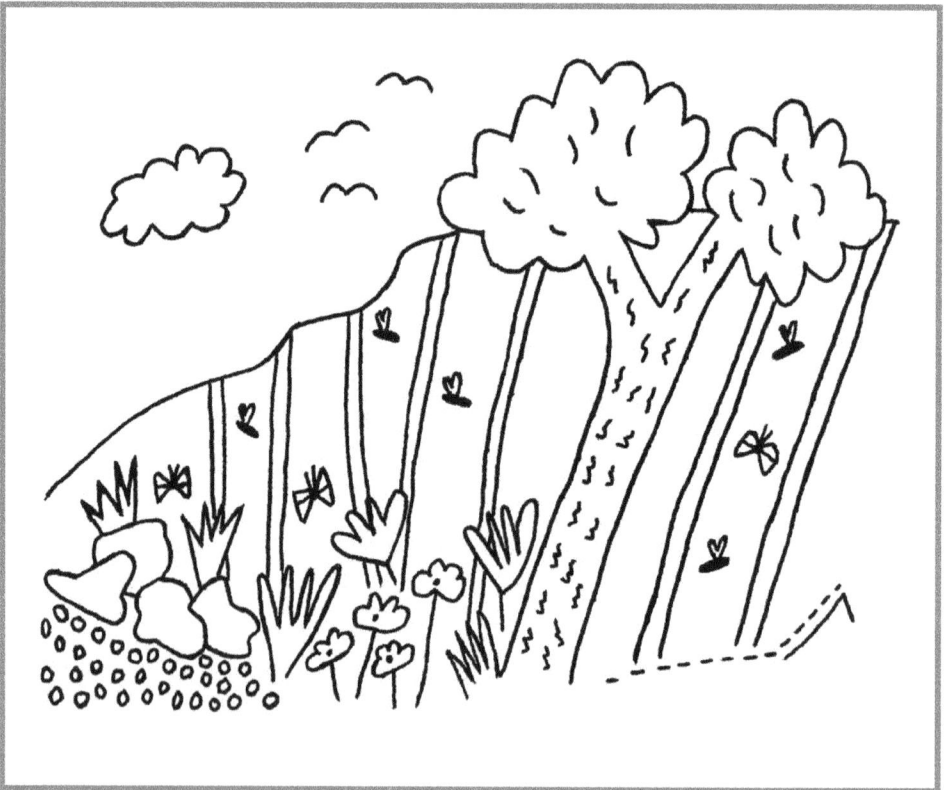

Reality Shows

- I like some reality shows, such as the singing competitions and the challenge shows. I don't like the love shows.
- I don't like soapies; I get bored with the bad acting and the social themes.
- When following my favourite reality shows, I will always have paper and pen ready to list all the stats such as the people, the challenges, the teams, and the eliminations.
- I am not interested in the social part of the shows.
- I love to study and memorise my stats and make up charts.

*Note : not actually one of my charts

name	challenge	food tasks	team	eliminated
Sam	✓✓✓	✓✓	blue	
Henry	✓		red	1
Mary		✓✓✓	blue	
Paula	✓✓✓✓		blue	
Harry	✓		red	
Tina	✓✓✓		red	
Janet	✓	✓	blue	2
Kevin	✓✓		blue	4
Larry	✓✓		red	
Stuart	✓✓	✓✓✓	red	
Sarah	✓✓		red	3
Cindy	✓✓✓✓	✓✓	blue	

Stuff in Order

- All my books are in alphabetical order by author.
- My music CDs are in alphabetical order by artist.
- My clothes are in colour order and category such as T shirts, going-out short sleeved tops, long sleeved tops, warm long sleeved tops (all in colour order).
- I have framed photo boards and near the boards is a small book which tells where every photo was taken.
- I collected stones during our Darwin trip and written on each stone is the location where it was found.

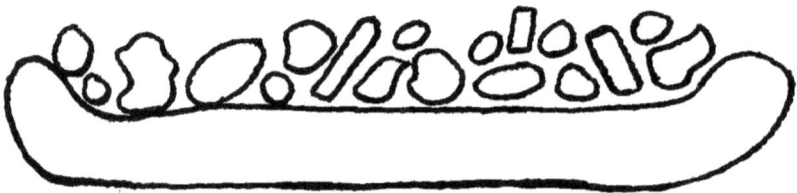

my stone collection

What I Love

- I love lots of things:
- I love my filing cabinet. All of my information is in easy-to-locate sections.
- Lego and Ikea (just big Lego) are so amazing. All those lovely steps and rules and you can build something astonishing.
- Details and patterns are so pleasing to look at, so much order and structure.
- I love learning new information, facts, and stats. Just right for my Google brain.
- I love to put information into charts and lists.
- I can organise huge messes and place items into categories. The bigger the mess, the better.
- Some words and sounds are really pleasing to my ears and I like to repeat them out loud to myself.
- To help me work things out, I love to compare information (black and white thinking). If it is not this, it is that. It makes life simpler to me.

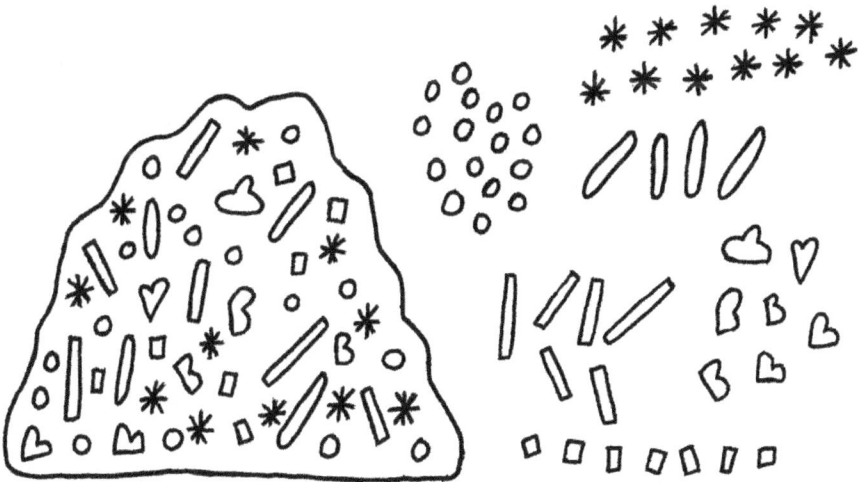

'I WASN'T THE ONLY ONE SPILLING MY GUTS'

16

ACHIEVEMENTS

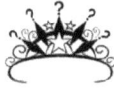

- Around Australia
- A Few Statistics
- Retire at 38
- Bibbulmun Track
- Rollercoaster

Around Australia

- Age: early 30's

- I have a one-track mind and the tenacity to conquer massive tasks. This includes travel planning, which I do in great detail.

- In 1999/2000 Oliver, Aaron (aged 5) and I travelled for five months to the east coast of Australia, going from Perth to central Australia, then to Queensland, New South Wales, Victoria, Tasmania, South Australia and then back home to Western Australia.

- To plan this big trip, I spent a whole year reading and making notes. Oliver researched bush safety, the camper and the four-wheel drive stuff, while I sat at the dining table and read and read. I stayed in the same spot and researched (no computer, just books). The rest of my life went on hold. Oliver fed me. This became the template for all our future travel planning.

- In 2004, when Aaron was ten, the three of us travelled for four months, going to Darwin and back home through Western Australia.

- During 2012 to 2014, Oliver and I spent one year and seven months travelling the whole of Australia: Perth to the northern part of Western Australia to the Northern Territory, South Australia, Victoria, Tasmania, New South Wales, Australian Capital Territory, Queensland, central Australia, then back through Western Australia and home to Perth.

- I read about all the country towns, National Parks, cities, tourism and interesting things in Australia. Then I got a map of each state we would be visiting and placed red dots on all my researched places. Next I drew a line to connect the dots. If something was too far from the line, I deleted it from our itinerary.

- I researched all the walks in the National Parks and printed out the park guides.

- I wrote up books with all 581 days worked out. I included rest days, washing and repair days.

- Everything worked out perfectly, all the days exactly as I planned.

Extract from my book

Day 565, 566 December 27, 28 Friday, Saturday	· Ruby Gap Nature Reserve	· walk – Glen Annie Gorge 8 km^s
85 km^s	Camp 2 nights	
Day 567, 568 December 29, 30 Sunday, Monday	· Arltunga Historical Reserve · Alice Springs	· walk – Government Works – Mac Donnell Mine – Joker Gorge 1km
182 km^s	Camp 2 nights	
Day 569 December 31 Tuesday	· Tennant Creek	
513 km^s	Camp	
Day 570, 571 January 1+2 Wednesday, Thurs.	· Daly Waters Pub · Katherine	· flight over Kakadu National Park
678 km^s	Camp 2 nights	
	· Nitmiluk National Park	· Walk – Edith Falls 2·6 km^s

165

A Few Statistics

- During our trip around Australia, we wore through two sets of tyres, three pairs of shoes and dropped two cameras in the water. We set up the camper 247 times and set up the tent 13 times.
- We took 40,000 photos and I reduced them down to 4,000. I made up 40 books with diary notes and photos.

- Time spent in each state:

WA	9 weeks + 1 day
NT	11 weeks + 6 days
SA	4 weeks + 2 days
VIC	11 weeks + 1 day
NSW	17 weeks + 4 days
QLD	20 weeks + 3 days
TAS	8 weeks + 4 days

- Total kilometres travelled: 73,322 kms
- Total kilometres walked (National Parks): 1,197 kms
- Hardest walk – Mount Augustus in Western Australia, a 12 km hike; it took 6 hours 25 minutes.
- Longest time in one place: Melbourne, 11 nights
- Most kilometres driven in one day: 678 kms, 1 January 2014

- Costs:

Repairs and maintenance to 4WD and camper	$ 20,839.84
Diesel and gas	$ 20,162.21
Accommodation	$ 25,325.01
Food	$ 33,400.11
Extras, shopping	$ 22,094.30
Excursions, entrance fees and ferry to Tasmania	$ 8,001.04
Total Costs:	$ 129,822.51

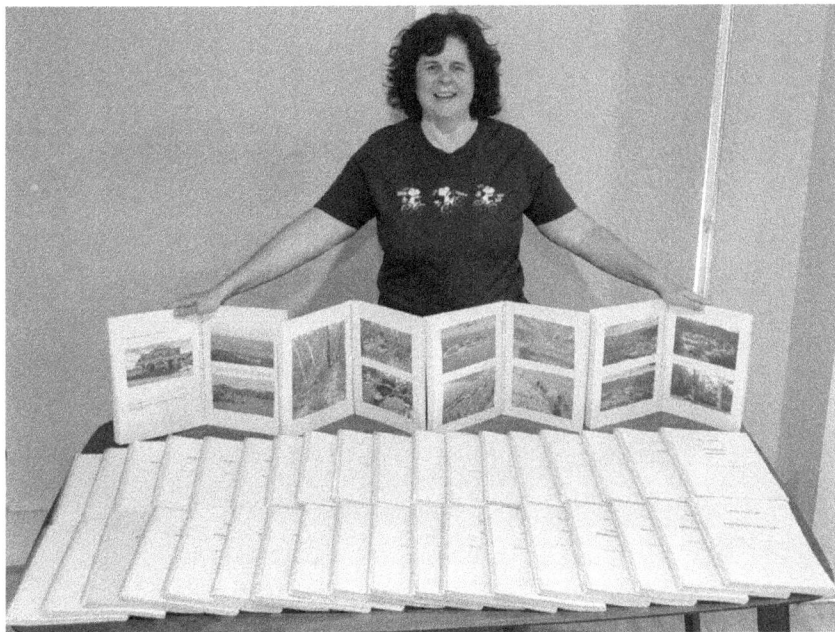

The 40 books

Retire at 38

- At age 22, I was looking for properties to buy. Then I met Oliver, and we bought our first two properties together.

- Two years later we sold those and bought our forever home.

- Ten years later, after our five-month holiday to the east coast of Australia, we were searching for financial freedom. I saw a real estate course advertised in the newspaper and I attended without Oliver (it was too expensive for both of us to go).

- There were about 750 people at the course. When the course was complete, I followed the advice given and we bought seven Perth properties in one and a half years.

- My Aspergian brain didn't worry about social but just followed the instructions.

- Three years later, at another wealth course, we met a guy, and we teamed up with him to buy properties in fifteen country towns.

- Properties consisted of vacant land, units, and houses.

- In 2004, I stopped working and Oliver stopped working two years later.

- I later learned that I was the only person from the 750 people at the initial course who bought properties. I had been panicking, thinking I had to compete with all these people buying properties. Oliver always trusted me, and I knew I had his support.

Bibbulmun Track

- Age: mid 50s

- The Bibbulmun Track is a hiking track covering 1,005 kilometres from Kalamunda (Perth) to Albany in the southwest of Western Australia. The track passes through nine country towns.

- We left on 31 August 2021 and arrived in Albany 67 days later on 5 November 2021.

- We hiked hut to hut (49 of them in total) and slept in them at night.

- Hiking the track was hard, very hard.

- You must carry a pack with everything in it, such as food, tent, cooker, clothes, technology, safety items and sleeping bag and mat.

- Our longest day was from Peaceful Bay to Boat Harbour which took 9 hours 15 minutes and included crossing a river by canoe. That day's hike was 23 kilometres long.

- There were 20 days of hiking more than 20 kilometres per day.

- We walked in all types of weather including hail and lots and lots of rain.

- The hike was over a huge array of terrain - hills (so many hills), valleys and flat areas. The hike went up every mountain available, mountains I didn't know even existed until we had to hike up and down them.

- There was a lot of walking through water, either through water crossings or swollen swamps, thigh deep at times (one swamp was over a kilometre long).

- The last kilometre to nearly every hut always seemed to be up an enormous hill and felt more like three kilometres.

- The Bibbulmun Track was our first long distance hike. Prior to this we had only done day hikes with our 4WD as our base.

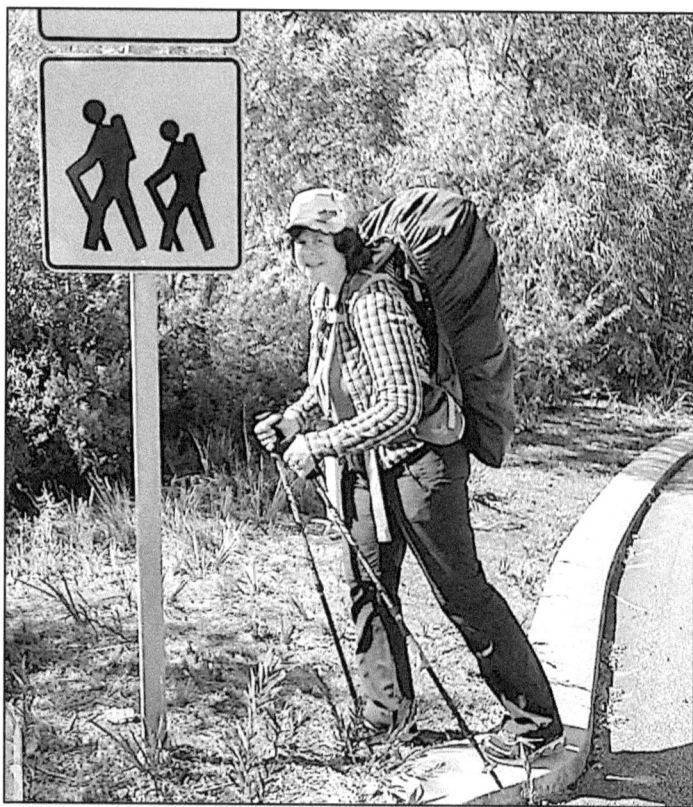

Following the rules

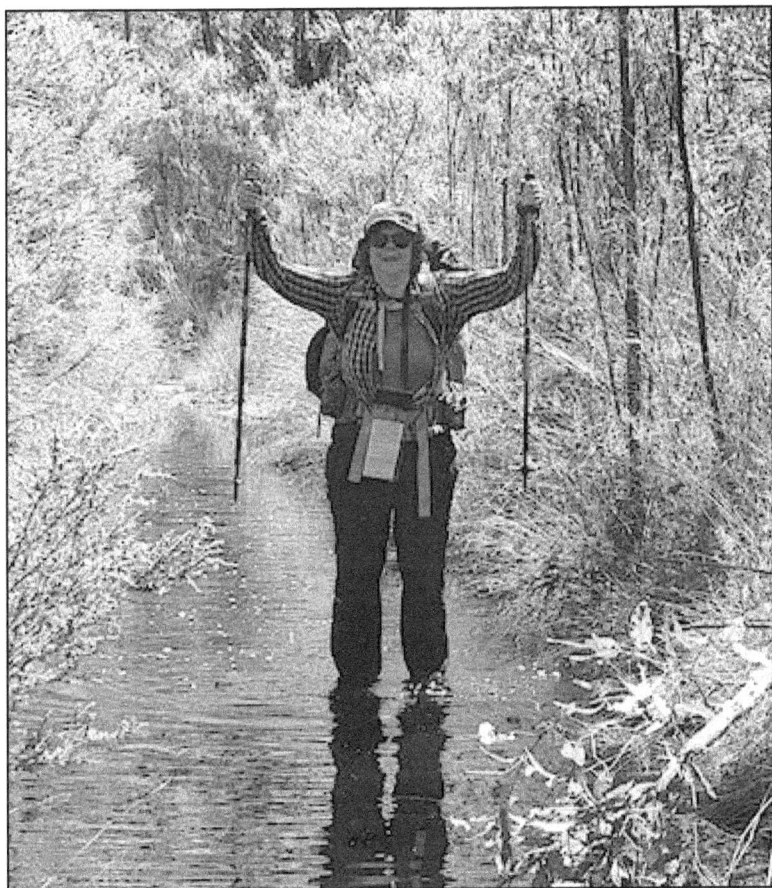

The water was fun

Rollercoaster

- We found the Bibbulmun hike so bloody difficult. I was in great pain with plantar fasciitis in both feet. I had a lot of tantrums.

- Oliver was always supportive. We were both too stubborn to give up - we wanted to push ourselves and conquer the challenge.

- We met some amazing fellow hikers. Everyone's emotions were on a rollercoaster ride. I soon found that I wasn't the only one 'spilling my guts' after another day of pushing ourselves to the edge.

- Gathered around the hut at night, people's social shields started to crumble because they were too exhausted to keep them up. It was quite an experience - watching people behave without their shields, just like me. When I first met Oliver, he was amazed that I would tell a total stranger all my secrets, and now everyone at camp was like me.

- Oliver and I did a lot of personal development whilst hiking. I learned patience and we both learned to be more peaceful and live in the 'Now', concentrating on the present; how you walk, moving your legs and arms, breathing.

- My pace is erratic - fast, slow and everything in between - so Oliver took the lead with his even, steady pace.

- Our love grew because we had to support each other so much.

- Afterward, we both agreed that long distance hiking was not for us.

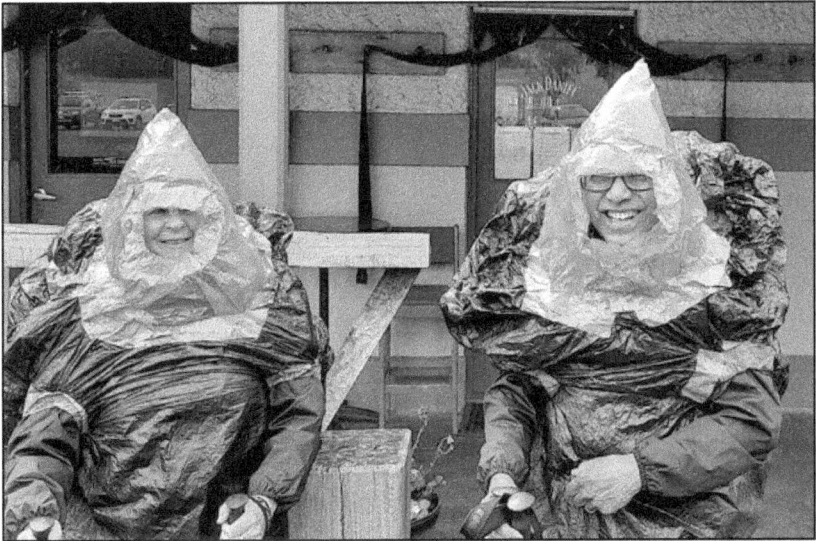

Our improvised rain gear

'MY IDEAS CAN LOOK WEIRD TO OTHERS'

17

MY WAY
(AND THAT'S OK WITH ME)

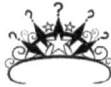

- Upside Down
- I'm OK
- Lovely Lynwood
- Oneness
- I Can Do Anything
- Fashion
- New Zealand

Upside Down

- I like to do things my way - solve problems with my logical brain and not be swayed by the general population. The way I solve problems can look unusual to others but it makes sense to me.
- When I was 11 years old I rode my bike to primary school every day.
- In winter, I was tired of my bike seat always being wet so I turned my bike upside down. Problem solved.
- The only catch was that when I went to my bike after school, my bike tyres were full of thumb tacks. But my seat was dry.
- I had to push my bike the 3 kilometres home.

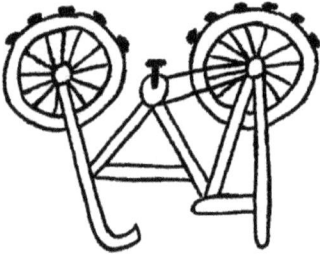

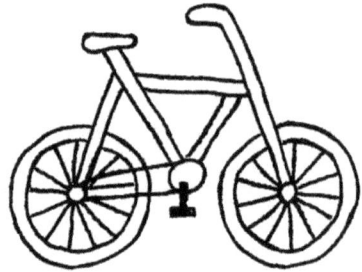

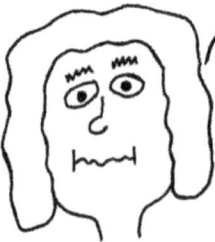

Thinking Back...
I still do things my way,
I just don't always make my ways public.

I'm OK

- Age: early 20s
- I was in central Perth and wanted to get home. I decided to walk. It was 10 kilometres. It was hard but I enjoyed it.
- When I got home, my flatmate yelled at me, 'Why didn't you ask me to pick you up?'
- Another situation occurred when I was working as a casual for a settlement office.
- My job was to go to appointments at banks and other settlement offices to exchange money and documents.
- One day, there were some appointments all at the same time. I just ran as fast as I could from office to office. Some settlements were cancelled because I wasn't there in time.
- Back in my office, the manager yelled at me, 'Why didn't you ask for help?'

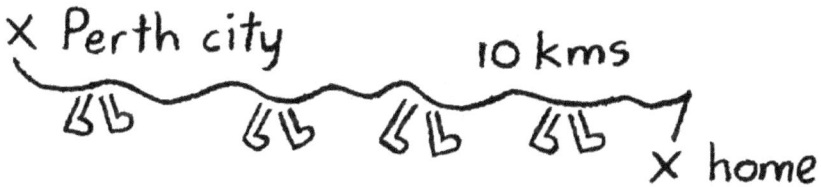

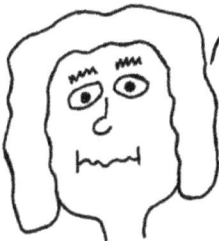

Thinking Back...
I did not know I could ask for help.
I just solved the problems my way.
Now I know I can ask others to help me.

Lovely Lynwood

- Age: early 20s
- I worked in East Perth and every evening after work, I would go on any bus into Perth city, then get off and walk to the Perth Central bus station.
- One night, the first bus turned and went down the freeway. I was pressing the bell, but the driver said he couldn't stop on the freeway, the next stop was Lynwood, 19 kilometres away.
- I stayed on the bus for the entire tour and was dropped off at the Causeway Bus Depot at 10.30 pm.
- I then walked past my work to try again to get home, five and a half hours later.

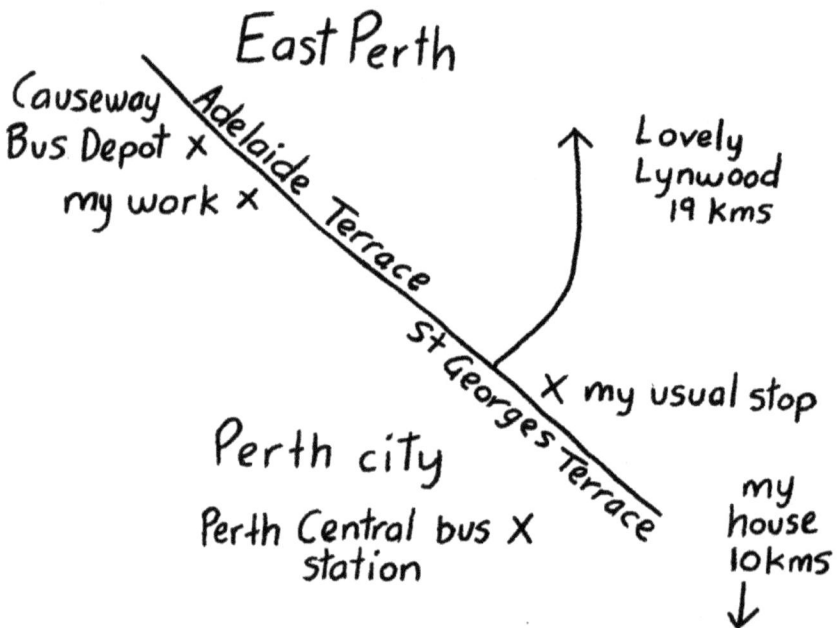

East Perth

Causeway Bus Depot X

Adelaide Terrace

my work X

Lovely Lynwood 19 kms

St Georges Terrace

X my usual stop

Perth city

Perth Central bus X station

my house 10kms

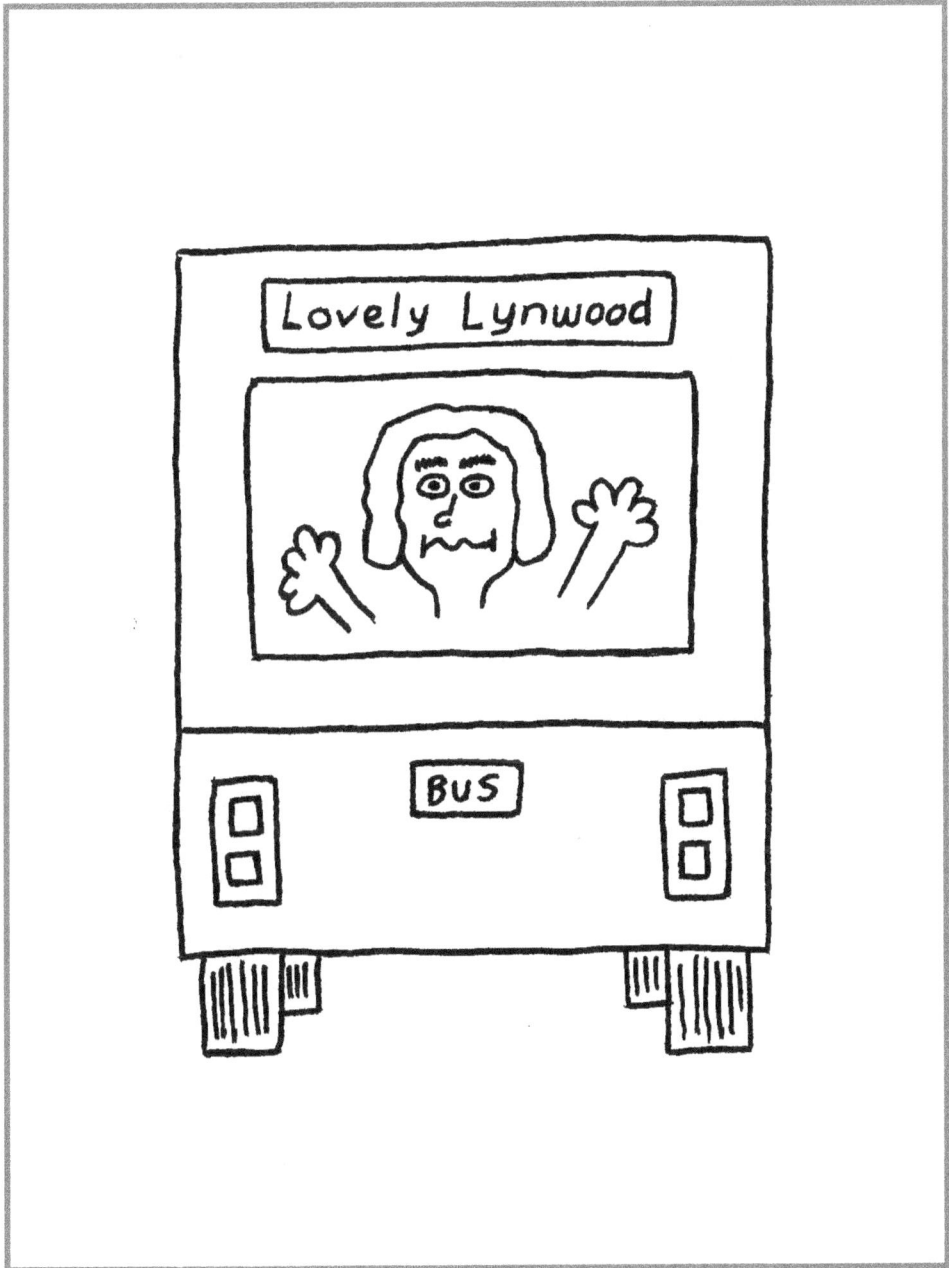

Oneness

- Oneness and social justice are very important for me.
- If everyone looks after each other, it spreads, and more people help others.
- My heart really goes out to people who display oneness, the real Aussie mateship, pitching in and helping a mate.
- Oneness has no ego involved. Ego is all about 'me, me, me'. Oneness is about everybody.
- One time I was waiting in the car while Oliver was in the shop. Three people, two guys and an older woman, went into the bottle shop. The two guys came out. They were laughing as they hopped into their car and drove away, knowing they had left the woman behind. The woman came out of the shop and realised her ride had left without her. I thought 'No way.' We put her in the car and drove her home. It was great to see the faces of the two guys (out the front of their house) when she arrived home. Their 'joke' didn't work with me.

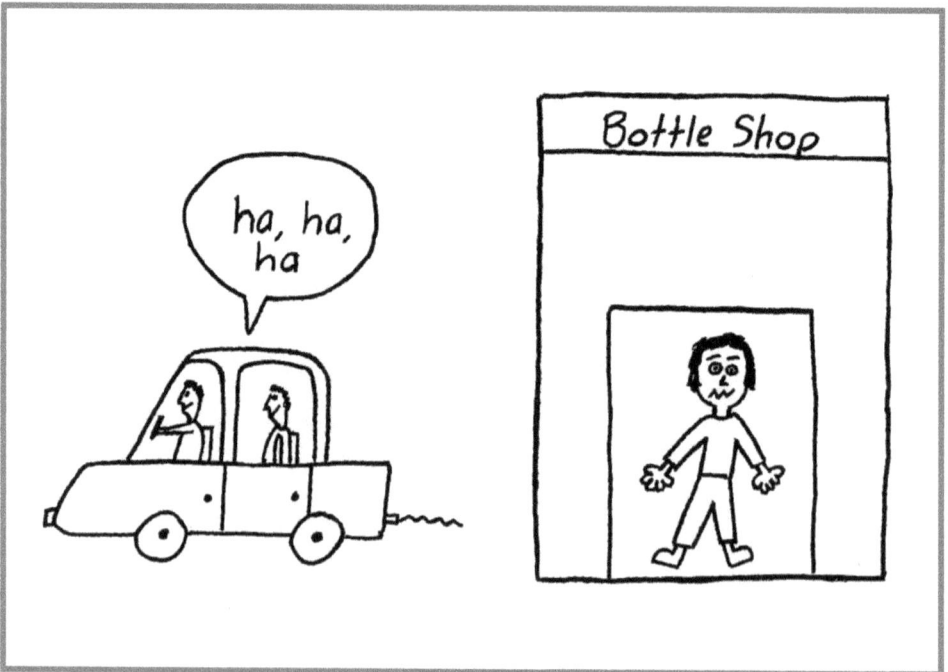

I Can Do Anything

- I have a tenacity to keep going until the task is over. I am single-minded and think about nothing else except the task at hand.
- Hierarchy is not important to me. I view people as individuals with different skills.
- I am really grateful that people study hard and become doctors and other kinds of skilled professionals.
- I am not socially attached to ideas. I like to get a person's opinion if they have true knowledge. My final decision comes from my gut, heart, and intuition – not from social information.
- My ideas can look weird to others but if they work for me and are logical, that is the answer.
- I can do anything; I am not scared to try new things.
- If something does not work, I learn from it.
- Sometimes I do things wrong on purpose because I like to try different ways.

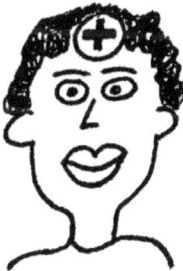 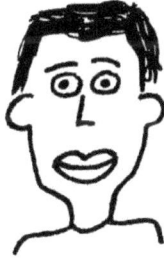 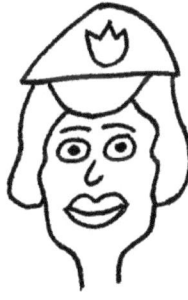 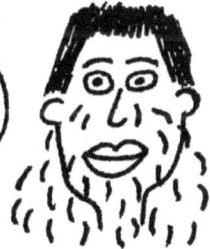

doctors   teachers   police   athletes

thank you

Fashion

- I don't follow fashion. I make my own fashion. These days I like jeans and colourful t-shirts.
- I have never owned a handbag. I like pants with big pockets. Handbags are not logical, all your important and valuable stuff in a 'ready to steal' bag.
- I like flat shoes; my legs are long enough.
- I have never known what to do with my hair. I like to just run my fingers through my hair, and I'm ready to go.
- I love socks. I like the feeling of my feet being 'cuddled'.
- I don't carry a phone with me. I own a phone but rarely look at it.

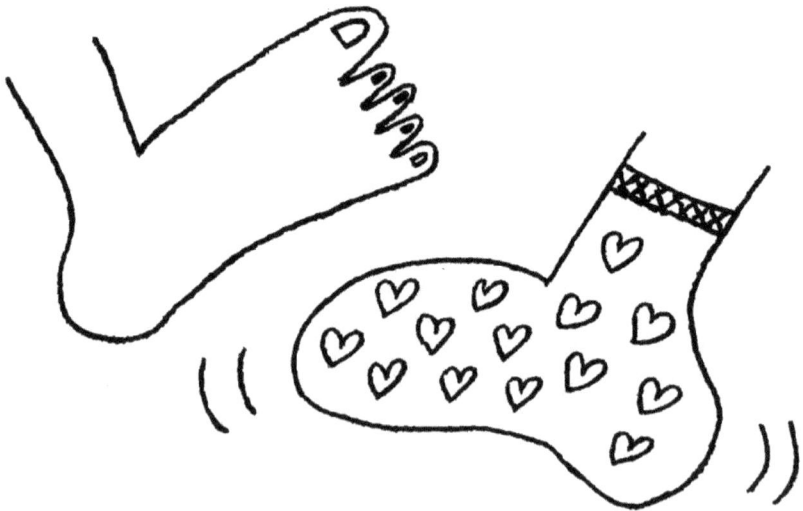

New Zealand

- Oliver, Aaron, and I went to New Zealand for a month.
- I was probably annoying Aaron, now a 15-year-old teenager, with bossing or rules.
- He was taking photos of me and Oliver and one day he made sure I was not in any photos.
- People are shocked when I tell them this story, but I thought it was so funny. I didn't worry about the social side, just the humour.

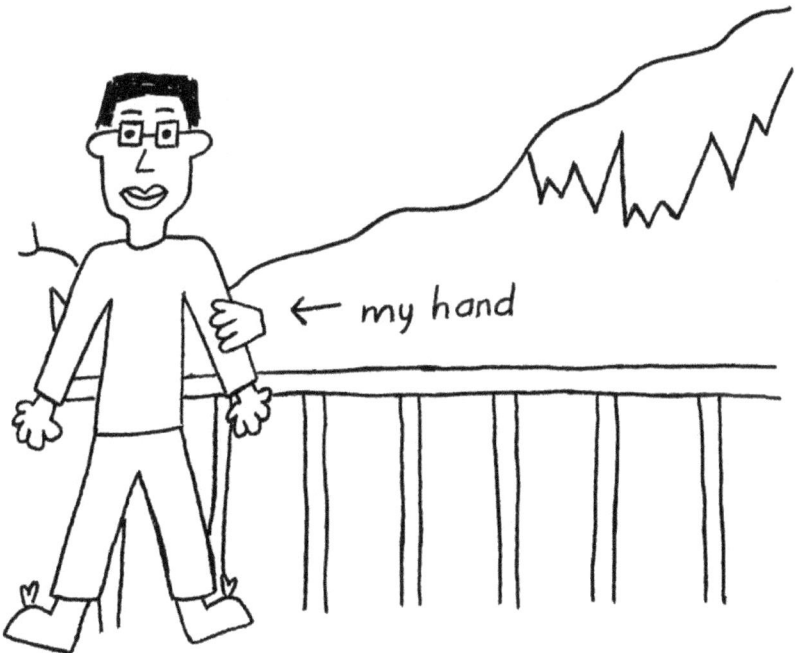

← my hand

'I HAVE BEEN WATCHING AND COPYING PEOPLE MY WHOLE LIFE'

18

COOL AND BEAUTIFUL

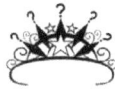

So Who Am I Now?

- Parents help you understand your strengths and weaknesses. They encourage you to believe in yourself and to become an independent person. They are proud of your achievements and want you to succeed.

- In an abusive childhood, the child doesn't develop an identity. You are kept as an object. The parents want to keep you small and totally dependent on them. You cannot cause any problems. You are not encouraged to shine. You are controlled with guilt, shame, and blame. You don't know who you are, you have no identity.

- I still struggle with identity.

- I have been watching and copying people my whole life and I feel like I act like someone else at times, like an impostor.

- I know that Oliver wears different hats. He has different behaviours for when he is at home with just Aaron and me, when he is with family, when he is with friends or around strangers. I act the same with everyone.

- I know I am a deep thinker and I probably want 'Meaning of Life' answers.

- I have tried to list my qualities but doesn't everybody have the same list? People just list what they think others want to hear, they lie and sound superficial, they say whatever the latest 'new identity' is at the time.

- When I try to think of my list, my mind and heart are empty, I just don't know.

- Aaron knows who he is because I told him his special qualities, he is an adult now and I still tell him.

- Aaron says I am cool, and Oliver says I am beautiful, so I'll just use that as my identity: Cool and Beautiful.

I'm Cool and Beautiful
I'll hug my inner queen, see my crown

Stand tall, I'll lift my head high
I'm proud of myself, my sparkly crown

I live by my own rules
I'm unique and special, see my crown

I'm Cool and Beautiful
I'll live in the 'Now', my sparkly crown

Virginia Sta Maria - 2025

ACKNOWLEDGEMENTS

After I wrote my manuscript, the first person I wanted to get feedback from was Dr. Winnie Yu Pow Blake. I sent her a copy and waited impatiently for one week before she replied. I was sitting in a café with Oliver and when I read her text reply, I was in tears; if she believed this book could be a success, well that was all I needed. I asked if she could write the foreword and without hesitation, Winnie said 'Yes.' I am blown away with appreciation because without Winnie's foreword, I would not have a book, there would not be any credibility. Thank you, Winnie, you are the 'Aspie Whisperer'.

The next person who read the manuscript was Helen McKerral, a friend I made on the Bibbulmun Track hike. Thank you, Helen, for your advice on getting an editor and to leave my emotions and ego out of the book editing process.

When I was having doubts about the direction of the book, I approached Dr. Jasmine McDonald. I knew Jasmine would give me no-nonsense, empowering advice. Thank you, Jasmine, your advice gave me strength and it worked.

I never went to university, so spending so much time at Curtin University made me feel special. At Curtin I met Professors Tele Tan, Torbjorn Falkmer and Marita Falkmer and was introduced to a neurodiverse world and found that I had information to share.

From the very first time I met Tele in 2014, I felt safe and accepted as I am. Thank you Tele for your genuine calmness. Your awareness level is amazing.

I always admired Torbjorn's confidence and knew any meeting he facilitated would run in a smooth and orderly fashion. Thank you Torbjorn for your 'dad jokes' which I always found funny and at times shocking.

When I first met Marita, I discovered such a warm, caring person. When I highlighted one of my Aspie struggles, I was amazed how fast Marita wanted to help me. Thank you, Marita, for your kind, respectful heart.

Speaking to Dr. Theresa Kidd, I felt she understood so clearly what it was like to be me and when she explained what other autistic people were doing, I thought 'Hey, I do that.' Thank you, Theresa, for showing me I am not alone.

Oliver has known Professor Aleksandar (Sasha) Janca for about 30 years, and he speaks so fondly of their intense talks. Thank you, Sasha, for your inquisitive mind, I love your questions which make me think and I love thinking.

To my son Aaron, I am the luckiest mama in the world. You have the most beautiful, kind soul of anyone I know. Thank you so much for helping me format my book from paper to computer and showing me how to digitise my illustrations. Thank you for reading every page and giving me helpful criticism. And the biggest, warmest thank you for allowing me to write about you. I have so much admiration and love for you because I know you only ever want to help others and if your stories can help people to learn what it is like living in a family like ours, that will give you so much joy.

For Oliver, I got so excited to show you each page as I wrote them and I know you laughed with me thinking 'Yep, that's Virg, that is just what she would do.' I love being married to you and know through the usual ups and downs of marriage that we stick by each other, and our love is stronger than ever. We have so much in common and I really enjoy all our adventures together, our deep conversations, our curious minds and our 'anything is possible' attitudes. Thank you Oly for allowing the world into our lives as a neurodiverse family. I know everyone will love you just like I do.

I would also like to thank my dogs, and yes, they have read my book - their favourite page is 'We Are Family'.

Lastly, in order of appearance, is Anna Johnson, my editor. I met Anna when she bought one of our outback properties. I knew she had written a book (Don't Try This at Home – Our Life in the Outback) and when I read it, I laughed so hard - her sense of humour is just like mine, so I knew she would be a great fit for me. I gave Anna a copy of my manuscript and she emailed back 'very powerful, brave, inspiring, fresh, funny, insightful and very moving.' Wow, wow, wow, wow. I was in Basic in English (the lowest class) at high school and here was an author giving me inspiring words for what I had written. I gave Anna free rein over my whole book because I trusted her wisdom. Every time Anna came back with another total edit, I was blown away with just how professional my book was becoming. She asked lots of questions, some very hard for me to answer, but I knew it was always for a better, clearer understanding of my world. A massive thank you Anna (through tears), you are so important and valuable to me. I have clearly won the lottery when you came on board to help me. And a final enormous thank you, bigger than the last thank you, thank you Anna for not changing the style of my book because the way I designed it shows my true authentic Aspie self.

Virginia Sta Maria

2025

ABOUT THE AUTHOR

Virginia Sta Maria lives in Perth, Western Australia. She is married with one son and two adult stepchildren and has been an advocate for neurodivergent people since 2014. She was part of the founding team for the Autism Academy for Software Quality Assurance (AASQA) at Curtin University, where she and her husband Oliver served as advisory board members for many years. Virginia was involved in the support and preservation of the Curtin Specialist Mentoring Program (CSMP), the university's neurodivergent mentoring program. With Oliver and their son, Aaron, Virginia was involved in many PhD research projects and twice invited as a guest speaker at the university's Autism Open Days. Virginia and Oliver were regular contributors to the Curtin Autism Research Group and the university's professional development sessions.

This is Virginia's first book. She plans to continue developing ways to support neurodivergent people and educate the non-neurodivergent by sharing her remarkable life experiences, achievements and humour.

For all enquiries regarding sales, events and publicity,
please email:

aspirationsautism@outlook.com

www.ingramcontent.com/pod-product-compliance
Lightning Source LLC
Chambersburg PA
CBHW050841270326
41930CB00019B/3425